The American Nurses Asso
organization representing tl
through its constituent/state nurses associations and its organizational affiliates. The
ANA advances the nursing profession by fostering high standards of nursing practice,
promoting the rights of nurses in the workplace, projecting a positive and realistic
view of nursing, and by lobbying the Congress and regulatory agencies on health care
issues affecting nurses and the public.

American Nurses Association
8515 Georgia Avenue, Suite 400
Silver Spring, MD 20910-3492
1-800-274-4ANA
http://www.Nursingworld.org

Copyright © 2021 ANA. All rights reserved. No part of this book may be reproduced
or used in any form or any means, electronic or mechanical, including photocopying
and recording, or by any information storage and retrieval system, without permission
in writing from the publisher.

Cataloging-in-Publication Data on file with the Library of Congress

ISBN-13: Print 978-1-947800-47-2   SAN: 851-3481
         ePDF 978-1-947800-48-9
         ePUB 978-1-947800-49-6
         Mobi 978-1-947800-50-2

First printing: January 2021

The Art and Science of
Nurse Coaching
2nd edition

The Provider's Guide to Coaching Scope and Competencies

By
Mary Elaine Southard, DNP, RN
Barbara M. Dossey, PhD, RN
Linda Bark, PhD, RN
Bonney Gulino Schaub, MS, RN

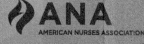

American Nurses Association
Silver Spring, Maryland

About the Authors

Mary Elaine Southard, DNP, RN, MSN, APHN-BC, HWNC-BC, DipHom, Chair
Executive Director and CEO, Integrative Health Consulting and Coaching, LLC
Founder, Nurse Coaching Community of Practice (NC-COPA)
Associate Editor, Journal of Holistic Nursing
Private Practice, Scranton, Pennsylvania

Barbara M. Dossey, PhD, RN, AHN-BC, FAAN, HWNC-BC
Co-Founder, International Nurse Coach Association,
Co-Founder and Director, International Communications,
Integrative Nurse Coach Academy, Surfside, Florida
International Co-Director, Nightingale Initiative for Global Health, Santa Fe,
New Mexico; Gatineau, Quebec; and Geneva, Switzerland

Linda Bark, PhD, RN, MCC, NC-BC, NBC-HWC
Founder and CEO, Wisdom of the Whole Coaching Academy,
San Francisco Bay Area, California
Principle and Chief Coaching Officer IM Health Diabetes Company,
Hopkinton, Massachusetts
Adjunct Coaching Faculty, California Institute of Integral Studies,
San Francisco, California
Faculty, Weljii Health and Wellness Institute, Delhi, India
Private Practice, Alameda, California and Black Mountain, North Carolina

Bonney Gulino Schaub, MS, RN, PMHCNS, NC-BC
Co-Founder, Huntington Meditation and Imagery Center
Founder/Director Transpersonal Nurse Coaching
Visiting Scholar, Texas Wesleyan University School of Health Professions,
Fort Worth, Texas
Private Practice
Huntington, New York

Contents

Authors and Peer Reviewers

The Art and Science of Nurse Coaching: The Provider's Guide to Coaching Scope and Competencies, 2nd edition, is the product of the authors along with a two-step review process of nurse coach experts and leaders. The review process included an expert panel review and a 45-day public comment period. This document is produced in collaboration with the American Holistic Nurses Association (AHNA) and the American Holistic Nurses Credentialing Corporation (AHNCC). The board certification for Nurse Coaching through AHNCC is accredited by the American Board of Nursing Specialty Certification (ABNSC) and Magnet recognized.

Professional Nurse Coaching Author Workgroup (2018–2020)

Mary Elaine Southard, DNP, MSN, RN, APHN-BC, HWNC-BC, DipHom (Chair)

Barbara M. Dossey, PhD, RN, AHN-BC, FAAN, HWNC-BC

Linda Bark, PhD, RN, MCC, NC-BC, NBC-HWC

Bonney Gulino Schaub, MS, RN, PMHCNS, NC-BC

Professional Nurse Coaching Review Committee

Karen Avino, EdD, RN, AHN-BC, HWNC-BC
Co-Founder and Director Education, Integrative Nurse Coach Academy, Surfside, Florida
Founder, Integrative Holistic Nursing Academy, Wilmington, Delaware

Janet Booth, MA, RN, NC-BC
Living Well Nurse Coaching,
Westcliffe, Colorado

Colleen Delaney, PhD, RN, AHN-BC, HWNC-BC
Associate Research Professor, University of Connecticut, School of Nursing,
Storrs, Connecticut

Deborah McElligott, DNP, ANP-BC, AHN-BC, HWNC-BC, CDE
Nurse Practitioner, Katz Institute, Center for Wellness and Integrative Medicine,
Northwell Health, Roslyn, New York
Clinical Assistant Professor, Zucker School of Medicine at Hofstra/Northwell,
Uniondale, New York

Amy Kenefick Moore, PhD, RN, CNM, FN, HWNC-BC
Associate Professor, University of Connecticut, School of Nursing,
Storrs, Connecticut

Heidi Ochtrup, BSN, NC-BC, CRN
Mayo Clinic,
Rochester, Minnesota

William E. Rosa, PhD, MBE, AHN-BC, HWNC-BC, FAANP, FAAN
Postdoctoral Research Fellow in Psycho-Oncology
Department of Psychiatry and Behavioral Sciences
Memorial Sloan Kettering Cancer Center, New York, NY, USA
Robert Wood Johnson Foundation Future of Nursing Scholar (2017–2020)
International Council of Nurses Global Nursing Leadership
Institute Scholar (2020)
Vice-Chair, Global Nursing and Health Expert Panel,
American Academy of Nursing (2020–2022)

Joanne Turnier, DNP, RN, ACNS-BC, HN-BC, HWNC-BC, CT
Integrative Healing Network,
Northport, New York
Adjunct Faculty St. Joseph's College,
Patchogue, New York

Heidi Taylor, PhD, RN, NC-BC, HN-BC
Dean and Professor, School of Health Professions, Texas Wesleyan University
Fort Worth, Texas

Catherine Winnell, BSN, RN, NC-BC, TNC
Private Practice Nurse Coach
Petoskey, Michigan

Toyoko Yasui, MSN, RN, OCN, AHN-BC, HWNC-BC, CCAP
Private Practice Nurse Coach
New York, New York

Acknowledgement

Special thanks to:

Erin E. Walpole, PMP, American Nurses Association, Editor/Project Manager

Carol J. Bickford, PhD, RN-BC, CPHIMS, FAMIA, FHIMSS, FAAN, American Nurses Association, Senior Policy Advisor

Terri Roberts, JD, RN, American Holistic Nurses Association (AHNA)

Margaret Erickson, PhD, RN, CNS, APHN-BC, American Holistic Nurses Credentialing Corporation (AHNCC)

Rebecca Lara, BS, Editor, AHNA *Beginnings*

Preamble

The health of the United States population ranks poorly compared to other developed countries even though healthcare costs are high (Foreman, 2018). More than 117 million Americans, almost half the adult population, live with at least one chronic disease (CDC, 2016). Besides people having poor health habits, U.S. healthcare systems lack effective ways to address the root causes of disease or to provide care that truly promotes health, well-being, and a high level of quality care. The major causes identified are as follows:

- Lack of engagement and disempowered healthcare consumers has been a reported issue for many years (Petri, Atanasova, & Kamin, 2017; WHO, 2009).

- Overprescribing of medication has been identified as contributing to serious health problems for the American public. Approximately 80% of the global supply is consumed in the United States, which has about 5% of the world population (Gusovsky, 2016).

- Medical errors are the third leading cause of death in the United States (Makary & Daniel, 2016).

- Lack of continuity and coordination of care (Jowsey et al., 2016).

Although current statistics and research findings reveal a dismal picture of U.S. health and health care, one of the future drivers for change is nurse coaching. The purpose of coaching is to empower and facilitate people in reaching their goals in order to improve their health and well-being.

Professional Registered Nurses (RNs) comprise the largest group of licensed health practitioners. Currently, there are 20.7 million nurses worldwide engaged in providing health care, with about 4 million nurses practicing throughout the United States (ANA, 2019).

There is a significant need for nurses to address the growing aging population and the increase in non-communicable diseases (NCD). These challenges require a more holistic and person-centered approach that is reflected in the philosophy and practice of nursing. Part of the World Health Organization's (WHO) global strategy is to mobilize political will to invest in building effective nursing and midwifery workforce development. The WHO High-Level Commission on Non-Communicable Diseases stated, "Within a multidisciplinary health workforce, nurses have especially crucial roles to play in health promotion and health literacy, and in the prevention and management of NCDs ... nurses are uniquely placed to act as effective practitioners, health coaches, spokespersons, and knowledge suppliers for patients and families throughout the life course" (Mechcatie, 2019).

The skills and competencies of nurse coaching have relevance in all nursing practice settings. Educating nurses to bring coaching skills into whatever setting they work will enhance the well-being of their patients, their colleagues, and themselves. This will also be of value to the healthcare systems that recognize and support this work. Nurses are unique in the vast scope of their presence within health care. Nurse coaching theory, philosophy, and practice place great value on presence and relationship with the patient.

Since the passage of the 2010 Patient Protection and Affordable Care Act, there has been a significant change in the way primary care is delivered (PPACA, 2010). This has resulted in the emergence of new roles for nurses that involve increased face-to-face management and care of patients. In a Robert Wood Johnson Foundation (2013) study of innovative approaches to primary care, nurses coordinated teams that worked in a variety of capacities. This included independent nurse visits in small, rural private practice settings as well as, transition management hospital visits and home visits. In this model, licensed RNs were practicing in a variety of roles, such as charge nurses, nurse care managers, and care coordinators, in addition to health coaching. This role included training in motivational interviewing. The RNs in this practice expressed a great deal of professional and personal satisfaction, which was derived from their high level of direct contact with patients. This was particularly so for those nurses practicing in communities where they lived (Flinter, Hsu, Cromp, Ladden, & Wagner, 2017).

Overview of the Content

Essential Documents of Professional Nurse Coaching

Professional nurse coaches practicing in the United States are guided by documents that assist in their professional decision-making. The American Nurses Association's *Code of Ethics for Nurses with Interpretive Statements* (ANA, 2015b), provides a framework for nurse coach ethical practice regardless of practice level or setting. Following the template of the American Nurses Association's (ANA, 2015a), *Nursing: Scope and Standards of Practice*, 3rd ed., this document presents a framework and context of nurse coaching practice and associated competencies that identify the evidence of standard of care. Expanding on the first edition of *The Art and Science of Nurse Coaching: The Provider's Guide to Coaching Scope and Competencies* (Hess et al., 2013), this document becomes the premier resource for professional nurse coaching practice for quality improvement, certification and credentialing, position descriptions and performance appraisals, educational coursework, and regulatory decision-making activities for boards of nursing.

For a better understanding of the history, content, and context related to nurse coaching, readers will find the additional content of the A–I appendices useful:

- Appendix A. *The Art and Science of Nurse Coaching: The Provider's Guide to Scope and Competencies* (1st editon, 2013)

- Appendix B. Selected Nurse Theorists that Align with Professional Nurse Coaching Practice

- Appendix C. Social Science Theories that Align with Professional Nurse Coaching Practice

- Appendix D. Interventions Frequently Used in Professional Nurse Coaching

- Appendix E. The American Holistic Nurses Credentialing Corporation (AHNCC) Nurse Coach Certification Process

- Appendix F. Global Health and Professional Nurse Coaching
- Appendix G. An Open Source EHR for Professional Nurse Coaching Practice
- Appendix H. Emerging Competencies for Graduate and Advanced Practice Nurse Coach
- Appendix I. Extant Nurse Coach and Nurse Coaching Literature Review

Audience for This Publication

Nurses working as coaches, in every clinical setting of practice, education, research, and healthcare policy, comprise the primary audience for this professional resource. Students, interprofessional colleagues, agencies, and industry will find this document an invaluable reference. In addition, individuals, families, groups, communities, and organizations can refer to this document to better understand nurse coaching practice and its impact within any healthcare setting and environment.

Function of Professional Nurse Coaching's Scope and Competencies of Practice

The contents of this document have been expanded and revised from the first edition, as new and broader patterns of knowledge, attitudes, and skills of the nurse coach role have been developed and accepted by the nursing profession. As with the first edition, the nurse coach role, scope of practice, tenets, and competencies have been subjected to formal periodic review and public comment prior to publication.

It is imperative to distinctly articulate the scope, characteristic competencies, and evolving boundaries of nurse coaching as other disciplines become involved in health and wellness coaching. Nursing, by definition, is a discipline dedicated to the "protection, promotion, and optimization of health and abilities; prevention of illness and injury; facilitation of healing; alleviation of suffering through the diagnosis and treatment of human response; and advocacy in the care of individuals, families, groups, communities, and populations" (ANA, 2015a, p. 7). The authority for nursing is based on a social responsibility, which is derived from a complex social base and social contract. Nursing's social contract reflects the longstanding core values and ethics of the profession, which provides grounding for healthcare in society. Nursing' has an obligation to advocate, assist, and respond to facilitate positive healthcare outcomes.

Basic, graduate, and advanced practice nurse coaches build on the competencies expected of registered nurses (RNs) by demonstrating a greater depth and breadth of knowledge, and by utilizing a unique subset and complexity of skills for nurse coaching. As nurses transition into the role of nurse coach, there is a definite paradigm shift that requires a more flexible and reflective way of thinking. The nurse sets aside the expert role and instead assists the person to identify and prioritize desired areas for change. Thus, goals originate from clarifying and identifying the person's agenda. While nurse coaches can continue to hold the role of educator, expert, care coordinator, and advocate, they utilize these coaching skills at the request and permission of the healthcare consumer. This, in turn, allows for greater active listening, masterful questions, direct feedback, presence, and partnership.

Function of the Scope of Practice Statement of Professional Nurse Coaching

The scope of nurse coaching practice describes the "who," "what," "where," "when," "why," and "how" of nurse coaching practice to provide a picture of the complex practice and unique skill set of nurse coaches. The scope of practice statement is accompanied by the competencies associated with the nursing process and the ANA Standards of Professional Practice for Nurses.

Function of the ANA Standards of Professional Practice

The American Nurses Association's *Nursing: Scope and Standards of Practice,* 3rd edition (ANA, 2015a), provides the organizational framework for professional nurse coach competencies. The ANA Standards of Practice and the Standards of Professional Performance are summarized in Table 1 for the convenience of the reader. The standards are authoritative statements of the duties that all nurses, including nurse coaches, are expected to perform competently regardless of role, or population, or specialty. Accompanying discussion of these standards are nursing theories, social science theories, and the International Coach Federation competencies (ICF, 2019). The six Standards of Practice (Table 1 left column) are standards that describe a competent level of nursing practice demonstrated by the critical thinking model known as the nursing process; the six nursing process components correspond to these standards. The 11 Standards of Professional Performance (Table 1 right column) are standards that describe a competent level of behavior in the professional nursing role appropriate to the nurse's education and position.

Function of the Nurse Coaching Competencies

New patterns of professional practice for nurse coaches and the associated competencies have been developed as the dynamic of nurse coaching practice has evolved. The list of nurse coach competencies is not exhaustive.

Table 1. ANA Standards of Professional Nursing Practice (ANA, 2015a)

Standards of Practice	Standards of Professional Performance
Standard 1. Assessment The registered nurse collects comprehensive data pertinent to the healthcare consumer's health and/or the situation.	**Standard 7. Ethics** The registered nurse practices ethically.
Standard 2. Diagnosis The registered nurse analyzes assessment data to determine actual or potential diagnoses, problems, and issues.	**Standard 8: Culturally Congruent Practice** The registered nurse practices in a manner that is congruent with cultural diversity and inclusion principles.
Standard 3. Outcomes Identification The registered nurse identifies expected outcomes for a plan individualized to the healthcare consumer or the situation.	**Standard 9. Communication** The registered nurse communicates effectively in a variety of formats in all areas of practice.
Standard 4. Planning The registered nurse develops a plan that prescribes strategies to attain expected, measurable outcomes.	**Standard 10. Collaboration** The registered nurse collaborates with the healthcare consumer and other key stakeholders in the conduct of nursing practice.
Standard 5. Implementation The registered nurse implements the identified plan.	**Standard 11. Leadership** The registered nurse leads within the professional practice setting and the profession.
Standard 6. Evaluation The registered nurse evaluates progress toward attainment of goals and outcomes.	**Standard 12. Education** The registered nurse seeks knowledge and competence that reflects current nursing practice and promotes futuristic thinking.
	Standard 13. Evidence-Based Practice and Research The registered nurse integrates evidence and research findings into practice.

	Standard 14. Quality of Practice The registered nurse contributes to quality nursing practice. **Standard 15. Professional Practice Evaluation** The registered nurse evaluates one's own and others' nursing practice. **Standard 16. Resource Utilization** The registered nurse utilizes appropriate resources to plan, provide, and sustain evidence-based nursing services that are safe, effective, and fiscally responsible. **Standard 17. Environmental Health** The registered nurse practices in an environmentally safe and healthy manner.

The competencies are periodically reviewed and revised based on the AHNCC's comprehensive Role Delineation Study (RDS), evidence-based research, adherence to evidence of standard of care, and acceptance by the nursing profession and the public. Emerging competencies for graduate and advanced practice levels for nurse coaching require further validation through research.

Application of the competencies is dependent on context. Whether the specifics of each competency apply depends upon the individual's purpose of the coaching interaction and the interventions provided. Mastery of competencies requires continual self-reflective practice and adherence to continuing education to expand knowledge, skills, and attitudes.

Professional Nurse Coaching Scope of Practice

Definition of a Professional Nurse Coach

The professional Nurse Coach is a registered nurse who integrates coaching competencies into any setting or specialty area of practice to facilitate a process of change or development that assists individuals or groups to realize their potential. Note: This document provides specifics related to the Professional Nurse Coach. For an easier read, "Nurse Coach" and "Professional Nurse Coach" will be used interchangeably throughout this document.

Definition of Professional Nurse Coaching

Professional nurse coaching is a skilled, purposeful, results-oriented, and structured relationship and person-centered interaction with a healthcare consumer that is provided by a baccalaureate-prepared or advanced practice registered nurse for the purpose of promoting achievement of a person's goals (Hess et al., 2013). Note: The word 'client' is used interchangeably with 'patient' throughout this document.

Achievement of the person's goals is accomplished by first establishing a co-creative partnership with the individual, acknowledging that they are the expert in their own care. The nurse sets aside the expert role and instead assists the person to identify and prioritize desired areas for change. Thus, goals originate from clarifying and identifying the person's agenda.

Overview of Professional Nurse Coaching Scope of Practice

The nurse coach role has roots in Florence Nightingale's legacy, nursing history, nursing theories, and the social sciences, honoring the individuals' needs, goals, and resources.

Grounded in holistic nursing theories and whole-person philosophy, this co-creative partnership honors the individual as the expert, while providing clarification and direction according to the person's agenda. Built on strengths rather than focusing on weakness, nurse coaching offers a safe space for an individual to explore resistance, barriers to healthier behaviors, and how to make changes that honor one's inner knowing and deepest wisdom. The professional nurse coaching practice:

- Incorporates both the *science* (critical thinking, use of evidence/research/theory [e.g., nursing theories, change theory including appreciative inquiry and motivational interviewing, coherence theory, resilience, complexity science, etc.] and *art* [e.g., intuition, creativity, presence, self-awareness assessment tools and practices, mindfulness, imagery, relaxation, music, etc.] of nursing practice).

- Includes the values and ethics of holism, caring, moral insight, dignity, integrity, competence, responsibility, accountability, and legality that underlie professional nursing.

- Incorporates culturally relevant philosophies and paradigms in a manner that promotes the achievement of person-centered goals.

- Recognizes that coaching interventions, inherent individual characteristics, cultural norms, and policies and systems influence healthcare consumer outcomes.

- Honors the relationship between the individual's internal and external environment in order to achieve optimal outcomes.

- Partners with the healthcare consumer to identify their agenda relative to achievement of their goals.

- Creates a safe environment for relationship and person-centered coaching that includes empathy, warmth, caring, compassion, authenticity, respect, trust, and humor if appropriate.

- Integrates professional nursing and coaching competencies to foster the achievement of the healthcare consumer's goals.

- Recognizes that self-reflection, self-development, and self-care are necessary to provide effective nurse coaching services.

- Values self in nurse coaching practice.

Evolution of Professional Nurse Coaching

Professional nurse coaching has gained significant recognition since its inception as a designated role within the profession of nursing. The momentum for the explosive growth of nurse coaching has many reasons. The increased fragmentation of care delivery and reimbursement has challenged healthcare leaders for innovative approaches to provide relationship and to create person-centered care. The global implication of nurse coaching resonates with culturally congruent care that empowers individuals, groups, communities, and populations to adhere to a commitment of health, wellness, and well-being.

The high cost of healthcare currently emphasizes value-based care as a priority that involves engagement from both providers and individual healthcare consumers. There is accountability for end outcomes, patient satisfaction, and patient participation in their plan of care. These components have influenced the healthcare landscape, leading to the professional development of nurse coaching to fully engage individuals, communities, and populations to facilitate behavior change and promote healthier lifestyle choices.

The nurse coaching framework and context for competencies follows the expectations of professional nursing practice. The American Holistic Nurses Credentialing Corporation (AHNCC) has developed and implemented a structure and process for a nationally accredited and recognized board certification in Nurse Coaching. This certification aligns with the requirements for an organization to achieve Magnet status recognition. The ANCC Magnet Recognition Program® provides a framework for practice that has significant impact for the evolution of nursing roles to demonstrate model components for transformational leadership, empowerment, professional practice, new knowledge, and empirical outcomes (ANCC, 2017).

Nurse coaching has become a valuable asset in relationship and person-centered healthcare delivery. The benefit of nurse coaching supports both cost and quality outcomes for the healthcare consumer. Nurse coaches may be employed by third-party payers and institutional organizations to support the overall care coordination process. Health and wellness programs, health maintenance organizations (HMOs), hospitals, and agencies that provide case management are increasingly employing nurses as health coaches to assist individuals in improving health outcomes. From point of care to administration, education, and management, nurse coaches are impacting healthcare in a positive way.

Integrating the Art and Science of Professional Nurse Coaching

Professional nurse coaches integrate their general and specialty nursing knowledge, skills, and competencies into all nurse coaching interactions. Nurse coaches focus on a shift toward health and wellbeing in clinical practice, education, research and healthcare policy. This focus will be explored throughout this book.

Note: To honor the many places where nurse coaches practice and serve others, the terms "healthcare consumer," "person(s)," "individual(s)," "group(s)," and "community/communities" are used interchangeably throughout this book.

The Who, What, and How of Professional Nurse Coaching

Who Is a Professional Nurse Coach?

Consumers of healthcare have acknowledged that working with a professional nurse coach "keeps them accountable" as well as supports them in a change process. From the healthcare consumer's perspective, this may be their first encounter with a medical professional who supports their overall strengths, lets them be the expert, and helps them identify their own resistance to change. Using inquiry and skillful communication, the nurse coach assists others to connect with their own internal motivation for personal change. The change process is grounded in an awareness that effective change evolves from within before it can be manifested and maintained externally. Negotiation and self-determination are central to the clarification of values, beliefs, and goals for the person to ultimately take action for health, wellness, and well-being.

The professional nurse coach works with the healthcare consumer, applying whole person-centered care principles and interventions that integrate biological, psychological, sociological, spiritual, cultural, and environmental dimensions.

The healthcare consumer is defined as the individual patient, family member, care provider, group, community, or population that is the focus of the coaching interaction. Therefore, professional nurse coaches are not limited to or defined by lifespan or disease condition parameters.

Professional nurse coaches are aware that disease and illness are often a result of detrimental social, economic, and political forces; thus, they recognized the social and environmental determinants of health (ODPHP, 2018). Following in Florence Nightingale's legacy to create healthy work environments, they recognize the social and environmental determinants that can be linked to a change in health status (Dossey, 2010). Social determinants of health include, but are not limited to, family composition, friends, religion, culture, race, gender, socioeconomic status, education, and occupation or profession. The environmental determinants of health include any external agent, food, biological, chemical, physical, social, or cultural factor that affects the health of individuals and communities. Nurse coaches are very aware of health disparity in underserved populations, and they address these issues.

Recognized as the most trusted professionals (Gallup, 2020), nurses are in the prime position to assist people toward sustained health and well-being. Their role in coaching healthcare consumers to achieve optimal health and well-being has a profound and far-reaching impact. Nurse coaches cultivate and motivate others; their mission is to instill confidence and to create cohesive teams and environments that lead to authentic, integrative healthcare in institutions, clinics, and communities (Horton-Deutsch & Anderson, 2018). Nurse coaches support the Triple/Quadruple Aim (Bodenheimer & Sinsky, 2014) recommended by the Institute for Healthcare Improvement (IHI, 2018). They offer specific strategies to promote and sustain health in a more comprehensive manner as demonstrated by partnering with consumers and interprofessional teams to offer supportive advocacy.

Nurse coaches are change agent leaders and engage in many interprofessional conversations about integrative healthcare. They thrive in environments that foster networking, change, collaboration, and an awareness of collective efforts to bring about integrative healthcare policy and healthcare transformation (Dossey, Luck, & Schaub, 2015).

Congruent with the mission and vision of the American Nurses Association's (ANA) Healthy Nurse, Healthy Nation™ "Grand Challenge" (HNHN, n.d.), nurse coaches recognize that their own self-care is an essential sustaining contribution to not only their individual lives but also to the overall health and well-being of all humanity (Beck, Dossey, & Rushton, 2019; Priani, Hong, & Chen, 2018). In healthcare, self-care is deliberate, self-initiated, and disciplined. It consists of evaluation, reflection, and nurturing so the nurse coach can be truly present.

What Is Professional Nurse Coaching?

Professional nurse coaching is a new proactive innovation for healthcare transformation (Erickson et al., 2016; Natschke, 2015). It differs from patient education by acknowledging healthcare consumers as experts in their own care. Assisting healthcare consumers to identify strengths to access their internal motivation for change is a process of inquiry and empowerment. This breaks the cycle of shame, blame, and failure. Many nurse theorists have recognized the importance of focusing on a person's strengths and resilience. For example, nursing theorist, Margaret Newman (1999) describes a new paradigm of health in which disease is not an "enemy" that strikes a "victim." Health and disease comprise a unitary whole of individual and environment (Newman, 1999).

As a new professional practice model, nurse coaching addresses performance, management, and clinical practice. When implemented in all healthcare settings, nurse coaching can facilitate evidence-based practice and provide measured outcomes, especially in the shift of healthcare delivery from acute care to community settings.

The nurse coaching lens acknowledges integrative, integral, and holistic philosophies and principles of the fundamental unity within and between all beings and their environments. Thus, nurse coaching includes the health and well-being of people everywhere that can be seen as a community (Rosa, Upvall, Beck, & Dossey, 2019).

Tenets Characteristic of Professional Nurse Coaching Practice

The following professional nurse coaching tenets are embedded in every competency in this document and are reflected in professional nurse coaching practice (Hess et al., 2013):

1. **The nurse coach's practice is individualized for the healthcare consumer.**

   The nurse coach encourages growth, wholeness, and well-being of the individual according to their values and cultural beliefs. They view every person as creative, resourceful, and whole. The nurse coach views the healthcare consumer as resourceful individuals with inherent answers and wisdom.

2. **The nurse coach establishes a coaching relationship with the healthcare consumer.**

   The nurse coach establishes a coaching relationship as foundational to the success of a coaching interaction. It is a relationship where the complexity of human experiences is valued. The nurse coach demonstrates unconditional positive regard for persons and accepts them where they are. Within the coaching relationship, it is understood that change is best achieved when aligned with the health consumer's goals, desires, and readiness for change.

3. **Human caring is central to nurse coaching practice.**

   The moral ideal of nurse coaching is grounded in the concept of human caring. The nurse coach brings one's entire self into the relationship with the whole self of the other person in order to protect her or his vulnerability, preserve her or his humanity and dignity, and reinforce the meaning and experience of oneness and unity.

4. **The nurse coach uses the nurse coaching process to guide nurse-healthcare consumer coaching interactions.**

   The nurse coaching process is a systematic and skilled practice that incorporates integrative, integral, and holistic approaches. The nursing process is expanded and reinterpreted to include widely used nursing theories and evidence-based social science theories and frameworks that redefine established concepts and terms. The nurse coach understands and adheres to professional and ethical standards that include providing respectful, compassionate, and culturally relevant integrative nursing care to all persons.

5. **The nurse coach recognizes the link between the internal and external environment of self and the healthcare consumer.**

   Nurse coaches facilitate and foster an authentic healing environment where all participants are valued, are respected, and can collectively explore their hopes and challenges. Using an integrative, integral, and holistic lens, nurse coaches assist with linking internal and external environmental factors and components to influence the person's movement toward growth, health, optimal functioning, and well-being.

The How of Professional Nurse Coaching

The "how" of nurse coaching practice is defined as the ways, means, methods, processes, and manner by which nurse coaches practice professionally. The ways in which nurse coaches practice reflect their philosophical, integrative, integral, and holistic worldview through a whole person-centered model of care. This addresses the biological, psychological, sociological, spiritual, cultural, and environmental aspects of health and well-being (Luck & Dossey, 2015). Nurse coaches walk with individuals through a self-discovery process and use nurse coaching competencies and patient engagement strategies to connect with individuals' strengths, meaning, and goals (Bark, 2011). Nurse coaches use a framework of the nursing process with a shift in terminology and content to create the nurse coaching process (see Nurse Coach Core Value 3). The interventions most frequently used in professional nurse coaching are listed in Appendix D. The depth to which nurse coaches use these interventions is determined by additional education, training, and certification.

The practice of nurse coaching is theory-guided and evidence-based using the latest information related to health, wellness, behavioral change and patient engagement. Nurse coaches translate the recognized patterns of knowing in nursing (i.e., personal, empirical, aesthetic, ethical, not knowing, sociopolitical) into their practice (see Appendix B). They participate in interprofessional collaboration and refer healthcare consumers to other healthcare professionals when needed.

The methods by which nurse coaches practice include the use of informatics, where available, in hospitals, clinics, and other healthcare settings. The use of electronic health records (EHRs) is valuable for practice documentation, continuous quality improvement, and clinical decision-making. Security measures are always implemented to protect the healthcare consumer's privacy and records.

The processes by which nurse coaches expand knowledge are to engage in research, develop protocols and guidelines, and implement strategies for greater health and well-being. Their research includes descriptive, explanatory, and exploratory designs. This may be achieved by qualitative, quantitative, and mixed methods, or other approaches (Taylor & McElligott, 2015).

Nurse coaches follow the American Nurses Association's *Code of Ethics for Nurses With Interpretive Statements* (ANA, 2015b), and follow directives of other governing and regulatory organizations and institutional review boards' protocols that guide professional nursing practice.

The Art of Professional Nurse Coaching

The nurse coaching core values and competencies guide professional nurse coaching practice, whether used with individuals, families, groups, or communities. At the heart of professional nurse coaching is growth of the whole person, that is the nurturing of an individual's biological–psychological–sociological–spiritual–cultural–environmental well-being. The nurse coach and healthcare consumer relationship is rooted in quality human caring, therapeutic presence, and deep listening (Southard, Bark, & Hess, 2016). The nurse coach brings their whole self into the coaching relationship with another or others. This relationship provides the person with a safe environment in which to express their feelings, goals, hopes, and dreams, and to share their vulnerability, pain, and suffering.

In the coaching relationship, there may be various shifts in consciousness, intrapersonal dynamics, and interpersonal relationships (Horton-Deutsch & Anderson, 2018). Many expressions of the lived experiences are shared through story (Delaney, Barrere, & Bark, 2020). Expressed as a sense of connection, unity, and oneness with another human, the story connects us to the larger environment, Cosmos, or Spirit, however defined. The story and lived experiences facilitate a flow of energy in the mind–body–spirit–culture–environment in the coaching relationship of each person. This may be manifested as anxiety, fear, frustration, creativity, coherence, resilience, or other emotions. Ideally, nurse coaches embody the following qualities (Dossey, Luck, and Schaub, 2015):

- Development of integrative, integral, and holistic perspectives that include biological–psychological–sociological–spiritual–cultural–environmental aspects of the nurse coach and the healthcare consumer;

- Recognition that self-healing is an ongoing process and necessitates intentionality;

- Willingness to model self-reflection, self-development, and self-care;
- Willingness to bear witness to one's own pain and suffering;
- Willingness to identify creative and self-defeating patterns in self;
- Willingness to bear witness to a healthcare consumer's and others' pain and suffering;
- Commitment to lifelong personal learning;
- Willingness to take responsibility for inner reactions to individuals and situations;
- Commitment to maintain a sense of presence, authenticity, and self-awareness in cultivation of a capacity for deep listening, mindful presence, and not knowing;
- Respect and love for the humanness of healthcare consumers and others;
- Commitment to creativity and innovation;
- Willingness to believe that change is possible for all;

The art of nurse coaching engages deep listening as a caring competency (Gelinas, 2018). The nurse coach attends to the individual's subjective experiences and internal frame of reference. The nurse coach views individuals as resourceful with inherent personal wisdom and insights. The individual chooses the topic(s) for coaching and determines the direction of the coaching session. There is no predetermined information or education to be offered, and there are no predetermined objectives or outcomes identified.

Nurse coaching recognizes and supports the individual's current way of being as they evolve and adapt toward desired changes and goals. The nurse coach spends time with the individual in discovery and acknowledges each person as expert in their own care. The nurse coach only moves into the nurse expert role, when indicated, to assist the person with situations such as personal safety or exploring incorrect information. The nurse coach remembers that "less is more" when it comes to coaching interactions. What needs to be shared emerges as the nurse "walks with the person" through a mindful discovery process (Gustin, 2018).

The nurse coach is curious and open, attending to the "present moment" and to what emerges. Nurse coaches pay careful attention to the thread of a person's story, patterns, perspectives, and reality while engaging in a free-flowing process of discovery. Nurse coaches trust their intuition regarding what to say or ask next instead of thinking about or pre-planning the next question. *They do not guide or lead the direction of the conversation, but instead honor the unique unfolding of each coaching session through caring presence.* Caring presence has been defined as "a holistic and reciprocal exchange between the nurse and the patient that involves a sincere connection and sharing of the human experience" (Dunlap, 2019). Actively listening with compassion and attentiveness, the nurse allows the story to unfold organically. In that unfolding, by skillfully using the "power of the pause," the nurse coach sets the example of being comfortable with silence. This gives space for the "aha" of discovery for the healthcare consumer to know what the next step will be.

The nurse coach conveys caring and compassion by asking powerful questions that are interspersed with authentic statements such as, "I see you," "I hear you," "I am walking with you," and "I am learning and understanding how you relate to the world and others." Some example questions include:

- Where do you want to be by the end of today's session?
- What do you want me to know most about you?
- What was one "pearl of insight" or takeaway for you from today's session?

As nurse coaches listen with intention and from a heart space, there is an unfolding and enfolding of the person's stories/narratives, history, experiences, and perceptions with new insights and possibilities. It is this space where transformative change to a "new me" often occurs (Dossey, 2015c; Goble, Knight, Burke, Carawan, & Wolever, 2017; Delaney, Bark, & Barrere, 2020).

Nurse coaches reflect on their own desires and motivations, remembering that the healthcare consumer is always the author of the story. Nurse coaching is a relational approach, and the boundaries of traditional decision-making models (describing the problem, elucidating conflicts, identifying principles, implementing solutions, etc.) often require more basic questions about the individual's experience, such as "What are you going through right now?" "What do you think is the best thing for you to do in this situation?" and "How might I better understand your experience?" (Dossey, 2015c).

The Science of Professional Nurse Coaching

Nurse coaching is a systematic and skilled process that is grounded in scholarly theory and evidence-based and evidence-informed professional nurse coaching practice. Nurse coaches are beginning to conduct new research to further their role (Dyess, Prestia, Marquit, & Newman, 2018; Dyess, Sherman, Opalinski, & Eggenberger, 2017; Frey & Ratliff, 2018; McElligott Eckkardt, Dossey, Luck & Eckardt, 2018; Ross et al., 2018; Stewart-Lord, Baillie, & Woods, 2018; Taylor & McElligott, 2015). Nurse coaches incorporate approaches to nursing practice that are integrative, integral, and holistic, and that include the work of numerous nurse theorists and scholars. Appendix B lists the most frequently used nursing theories. Appendix C lists other related social science theories and concepts commonly utilized in nurse coaching practice.

Philosophical Principles of Professional Nurse Coaching

Professional nurse coaches express, contribute to, and promote the understanding of the philosophy of nurse coaching that values healing. It also recognizes the four components commonly known as the metaparadigm in nursing theory—nurse, person, health, and environment (society) (Fawcett, 1995). The paradigms and worldviews of nurse coaches impact their nurse coaching practice as they reflect on the nature of human beings, health, environment, and caring.

Metaparadigm definitions may vary in different nursing theories; however, the four domains are seen as interrelated and interdependent, and each informs and influences the others. The metaparadigm components bring nurse coaches into the full expression of being present in the moment with self and individuals, and in all of their knowing, doing, and being that are briefly described next.

Nurse

- A registered nurse in the 21st century is in "service" to humanity through nursing, social action, and advocacy.

- The nurse is an instrument in the healing process where the nurse brings one's whole self into relationship to the whole self of another, a group, or with significant others.

- The nurse participates with other and reinforces the meaning and experience of oneness and unity.

- The nurse recognizes and implements integrative, integral, and holistic philosophies and practices in daily life and all professional endeavors. This creates the space for compassion, caring, unconditional presence, and authenticity to facilitate healing in self and others and to assist in recovery from illness or with transition into peaceful dying.

Person

- Each person is an expression of wholeness and unity, and is interconnected.

- Each person has the capacity to find purpose and meaning in life, and in different circumstances.

- Each person (healthcare consumer, family member, significant others, group, community, population) engages with a nurse in a manner that is respectful of a person's subjective experiences about health, health issues, health beliefs, culture, values, sexual orientation, and personal preferences.

- Each person shapes basic assumptions and worldviews about well-being and sees death as a natural process.

Health

- Health is a state or process defined by an individual in which one experiences a sense of growth, well-being, harmony, and unity.

- Health places the individual at the center of care and addresses the biological–psychological–sociological–spiritual–cultural–environmental aspects that influence one's healing and health and how to live with a disease, illness, and symptoms.

- Health of all people includes achieving equity and reducing disparities and barriers to healthcare.

- Health is a basic human right of the global commons and a bridge across boundaries and a path to world peace.

Practice

- Professional nurse coaching practice is both an art and a science, which integrates theory, critical thinking, critical reasoning, and evidence-based and evidence-informed practice.

- The values and ethics of caring, holism, dignity, respect, and integrity are woven into the nurse coach and healthcare consumer relationship.

- There are various philosophies, worldviews, and paradigms of health, wellness, well-being, healing, illness, and culture that must be understood and translated into the co-creative nurse coaching process to achieve healthcare consumer outcomes.

- Professional nurse coaching practice also includes advocacy, public policy, social justice, and healthcare delivery that will have a positive impact on society.

Environment (Society)

- Environment (society) includes both interior and exterior space.

- The interior environment includes the individual's feelings such as purpose, meaning, and mental, emotional, cultural, and spiritual dimensions.

- The person's physiology and inner knowing is the interior (internal) environment of the exterior self.

- The exterior environment includes external objects that can be seen and measured and can impact physical, mental, emotional, social, cultural or spiritual domains.

- Environment is redefined to include the planet, its natural resources and processes, and all species and living creatures.

- Nurse coaches facilitate the co-creative nurse coaching process with healthcare consumers to discover their goals, needs, and possibilities, and to access their personal wisdom.

- Nurse coaches participate as an instrument of healing by using caring, presence, trust, respect, authenticity, and intention.

- Nurse coaches integrate conventional and caring-healing modalities that facilitate biological–psychological–sociological–spiritual–cultural–environmental connections to deepen wholeness and unity.

- Nurse coaches engage in collaborative practice with other interprofessional providers within the community to strengthen partnerships and alliances while honoring all contributions.

Professional Nurse Coach Core Values: Integrating the Art and Science

Professional nurse coaches understand that the role, scope of practice, and competencies are linked to each of the American Nurses Association's six Standards of Practice and 11 Standards of Professional Performance (ANA, 2015a). The professional nurse coach's role is based upon the following five core values:

Core Value 1. Nurse Coach Philosophy, Theories, and Ethics

Core Value 2. Nurse Coach Self-Reflection, Self-Development, and Self-Care

Core Value 3. Nurse Coaching Process

Core Value 4. Nurse Coach Communication, Therapeutic Relationships, Healing Environments, and Cultural Care

Core Value 5. Nurse Coach Education and Research

These nurse coach core values and the nurse coaching competencies are aligned with the ANA (2015a) *Nursing: Scope and Standards of Practice*, 3rd edition, and the AHNA and ANA (2019) *Holistic Nursing: Scope and Standards of Practice*, 3rd edition, which are the foundation for nurse coaching practice, education, curriculum development, research, and healthcare policy. They are also foundational for the nationally recognized AHNCC (n.d.) Nurse Coach Certification process that has Magnet recognition (See Appendix E) and is grounded in role delineation tasks critical for competent job performance.

Core Value 1. Nurse Coach Philosophy, Theories, and Ethics

Nurse Coach Philosophy

The professional nurse coach's holistic philosophy shapes the "who," "why," and "where" of nurse coaching practice. It weaves together the threads of healing of people and the planet—local to global (Rosa, 2017).

Healing is a lifelong journey of seeking harmony and balance in one's own life and in family, community, and global relations (Dossey, 2016). Healing involves the physical, mental, social, and spiritual processes of recovery, repair, renewal, and transformation. This can lead to an increase in wholeness and often (though not invariably) order and coherence. Healing is an emergent process of the whole system, bringing together aspects of one's self and the body–mind–spirit–environment–culture–society at deeper levels of inner knowing. This process leads toward integration and balance, with each aspect having equal importance and value (Quinn, 2016). Healing is a sense of contentment and of freedom from struggle. This may lead to more complex levels of personal understanding and meaning, and may be synchronous, but not synonymous, with curing (Schaub, 2015).

Nurse coaches develop their capacities for healing intention (Bark, 2011). This is the conscious awareness of being in the present moment to help facilitate the healing process; it is a volitional act of unconditional love. Nurse coaches recognize that the healing process is a continual journey of changing and evolving one's self through life. It is characterized by the awareness of patterns that either support, challenge, or obstruct health and healing (Schaub, 2015). This journey may be done alone or within a healing community. Using multiple interventions and comfort care, the healing process may occur until a person's final breath (Hope & Rosa, 2018; Rosa, Hope, & Matso, 2018).

Nurse coaches facilitate healing relationships in their practice. They are aware that the quality and characteristics of interactions between two people allow for more harmony and balance. These interactions may involve empathy, caring, love, warmth, trust, confidence, credibility, competence, honesty, courtesy, respect, sharing expectations, and a heart-to-heart connection (Horton-Deutsch & Anderson, 2018).

The nurse coach's philosophy includes evolving one's own state of consciousness to higher levels of personal and collective understanding of both interior and exterior experiences. This acknowledges interior and exterior experiences with others where authentic power is recognized within each person—local to global (Dossey, 2016; Ross et al., 2018). Disease and illness at the physical level may manifest for many reasons and variables (Luck, 2015a; Luck, 2015b; Luck & Dossey, 2015). It is important not to equate physical health, mental health, and spiritual health. They are different facets of the whole jewel of health that involves recovery, repair, renewal, and transformation (Dossey, 2016).

Nursing Theories

Nurse coaching is theory guided, evidence based, and evidence informed. Nurse coaching philosophy evolves from many nursing philosophies (meaning of nursing phenomenon), grand theories (proposing a testable action), conceptual models (distinct frame of reference), and middle-range theories (specific precise focus). Each nurse coach chooses from among one or more nursing theories as the framework for their practice. The following list includes some of the nursing theories and conceptual models that support nurse coaching practice. While this list is not exhaustive, it highlights the most frequently used examples within different models of practice. Appendix B provides a brief overview of each of these nursing theorists and their conceptual models and theories, which are listed in chronological order of first publication:

Conceptual Models and Grand Theories in the Integrative–Interactive Paradigm

Roy—*Roy Adaptation Model*

Neuman—*Neuman Systems Model*

Orem—*Self-Care Deficit Nursing Theory*

Erickson, Tomlin, and Swain—*Theory of Modeling and Role-Modeling*

Dossey—*Theory of Integral Nursing*

Conceptual Models and Grand Theories in the Unitary-Transformative Paradigm

Rogers—*Theory of Science of Unitary Human Beings*

Parse—*Theory of Human Becoming*

Newman—*Health as Expanding Consciousness Theory*

Cowling—*Unitary Knowing in Nursing Practice*

Grand Theories About Care or Caring Paradigm

Leininger—*Theory of Transcultural Nursing*

Watson—Theory of Transpersonal Caring/Unitary Caring Science

Middle-Range Theories

Peplau—*Theory of Interpersonal Relations*

Barrett—*Knowing Participation in Change Theory*

Mishel—*Theory of Uncertainty in Illness*

Smith—*Theory of Unitary Caring*

Smith and Leihr—*Story Theory*

Cowling—*Unitary Appreciative Inquiry*

Resnick—*Theory of Self-Efficacy*

Dossey, Luck, and Schaub—*Theory of Integrative Nurse Coaching*

Social Science Theories

Appendix C provides a brief description of these social science theories. The most frequently used social science theories in nurse coaching are as follows:

Appreciative Inquiry—Cooperrider and Whitney

Complexity Science—multiple theories and theorists

Five Structures of Integral Consciousness—Gebser

Self-Determination Theory—Ryan & Deci

Health Belief Model—Becker

Immunity to Change—Kegan and Lahey

Motivational Interviewing—Miller and Rollnick

Positive Psychology—Seligman and Csikszentmihalyi

Psychosynthesis—Assagioli

Transpersonal Psychology—Grof

Transtheoretical Model Stages of Change—Prochaska and DiClemente

Reflective Practice—Johns

Resilience—multiple theorists

Sense-of-Coherence Theory—Antonovsky

Self-Efficacy—Bandura

Vulnerability Model—Schaub and Schaub

Nurse Coaching Ethics

The *Code of Ethics for Nurses with Interpretive Statements* (ANA, 2015b), serves as the ethical framework for nurse coaches and nurse coaching regardless of practice setting or role, and provides guidance for the future. *The Guide to the Code of Ethics for Nurses with Interpretive Statements: Development, Interpretation, and Application,* 2nd edition (Fowler, 2015), provides additional resources. These nine provisions explicate key ethical concepts and actions for nurse coaches in all settings. Each of the following nine provisions starts with the ANA descriptive statement followed by a description of how nurse coaches translate each provision.

Provision I. The nurse practices with compassion and respect for the inherent dignity, worth, and unique attributes of every person.

The nurse coach uses compassion and respectful communication by listening to the uniqueness of each person's stories from a whole-person perspective. This demonstrates integrative, integral, and holistic care, while modeling the inherent dignity, worth, and unique attributes of every person. Nurse coaches strive to maximize the good (autonomy, comfort, dignity, quality of life) and minimize the bad (pain, suffering).

The nurse coach and healthcare consumer relationship is built on deep trust, which can take time. Understanding the cultural beliefs in relation to health may inform the coaching process. These interactions honor the patient's right to dignity, self-determination, and independence. The nurse coach integrates whole-person care for each individual (family, group, community, population) where cultural beliefs, religion, spiritual beliefs, sexual orientation, socio-economic status, race, and age are respected. This also includes the inherent interconnectedness and worth of all species and ecosystems of the world.

Provision 2. The nurse's primary commitment is to the patient, whether an individual, family, group, community, or population.

The nurse coach aligns their professional practice with this provision. The reality of this commitment also includes awareness of planetary health as we live in the globalization of the world. A healthcare consumer's experiences of belonging to a group and the group's support are respected. The nurse coach places the individual at the center of care in which the healthcare consumer chooses the topics for the coaching session. The nurse coach co-facilitates the session by deep listening and helping the individual to hear new threads for her/his story that leads to goal setting and care planning. The nurse coach recognizes their own personal and professional biases and prejudices when coaching and creates time to discuss these challenges with one or more colleagues. Professional collaboration is essential in some situations. The nurse coach sets professional boundaries and refers individuals to other interprofessionals when needed.

The nurse coach interventions bear witness to, identify, and contribute to unity; they are not performed for the sake of law, precedent, or social norms. When nurse coaches fully engage with individuals, this evokes a capacity to connect to and be with another in an intersubjective, mutual, and authentic manner while honoring complexity and ambiguity. Nurse coaches view healthcare consumers, others, and society from a unitary and integral wholeness that reflects the fundamental values of a person-centered, integrative, integral, and holistic relationship.

Provision 3. The nurse promotes, advocates for, and protects the rights, health, and safety of the patient.

The nurse coach adheres to this provision and protects the individual's rights of privacy and confidentiality. If the nurse coach believes that the person would benefit from more information that is outside her/his scope of practice, a discussion with another provider would occur only if there is mutual agreement with the person being coached. At that time, the nurse coach communicates only what is necessary to share with other professionals. If healthcare consumers are worried about being participants in research studies, the nurse coach will explore the concerns with the person and assist them in ways to honor their beliefs and values before research participation. Promoting and protecting the health of patients speak to the voice of advocacy that is necessary in today's complex healthcare environment.

The nurse coach is very alert to a healthcare consumer's safety. Assessing a person's environment includes determining if there is fear of abuse or violence. They have the duty to report any concern of danger to self or others to the appropriate authorities. The nurse coach continues to address performance standards and review mechanisms so that their nurse coaching practice moves from basic to advanced knowledge and competencies integration. This focus also includes educating, advocating, and being an environmental activist by helping to implement not only workplace safety but also healthcare and public policies to support health and healing for individuals, the planet, and all ecosystems.

Provision 4. The nurse has authority, accountability, and responsibility for nursing practice; makes decisions; and takes action consistent with the obligation to promote health and to provide optimal care.

The nurse coach is a healthcare leader who embodies strengths, purpose, values, ethics, and vision that hold to present and future expectations of professional conduct. This includes opening to intuitive insights and inner wisdom, which allows for compassion, caring, empathy, purpose, authenticity, humility, and integrity to manifest.

Nurse coaches follow their state nurse practice acts, regulations, and guidelines. They do not practice across state lines unless they have an Enhanced Nurse Licensure Compact (eNLC) license that allows for coaching healthcare consumers in other compact states (NCSBN, n.d.). They participate in interprofessional endeavors to engage in the health of the environment—local to global.

Provision 5. The nurse owes the same duties to self as to others, including the responsibility to promote health and safety, preserve wholeness of character and integrity, maintain competence, and continue personal and professional growth.

The professional nurse coach models authenticity that is seen in the consistency of their beliefs, values, and actions. Nurse coaches strive for an embodied awareness of being mindful and conscious of the present moment as change takes place in the present. They are aware that personal and professional abuse and bullying must never be tolerated.

Nurse coaches are committed to lifelong learning to enhance nurse coaching knowledge, praxis, and competencies. Nurse coaches are leaders, and they expand their visibility in how to create a culture of health and well-being within healthcare in hospitals, clinics, communities, organizations, and corporations in our interconnected world.

Provision 6. The nurse, through individual and collective effort, establishes, maintains, and improves the ethical environment of the work settings and conditions of employment that are conducive to safe, quality healthcare.

The nurse coach has a moral obligation to help correct unhealthy and unethical healthcare environments within practice, education, research, and healthcare policy. This also includes a commitment to social and environmental inequities, and to strive for peace, justice, and strong institutions.

Provision 7. The nurse, in all roles and settings, advances the profession through research and scholarly inquiry, professional standards development, and the generation of both nursing and health policy.

The nurse coach's contributions to the profession are focused on developing, maintaining, and implementing the scope, and competencies of professional nurse coaching practice in conjunction with the standards of professional nursing practice. The nurse coach translates health ethics and the social and environmental determinants of health into practice, education, research, and healthcare policy. Nurse coaches include other key stakeholders to improve health and healing environments and health outcomes that will support a healthy planet. For example, they should inform local, national, and global policymakers about climate change that impacts personal and planetary health. Scholarly inquiry for nurse coaching is important for evidence-based best practice and advancement of the field.

Provision 8. The nurse collaborates with other health professionals and the public to protect human rights, promote health diplomacy, and reduce health disparities.

The nurse coach views health as a universal right. Nurse coaches have the obligation to advance health and human rights and reduce disparities. They engage in interprofessional collaboration and with concerned citizens to protect health, human rights, and health diplomacy, in many different situations that are often complex, are extreme, or occur in extraordinary practice settings that include many diverse communities.

Provision 9. The profession of nursing, collectively through its professional organizations, must articulate nursing values, maintain the integrity of the profession, and integrate principles of social justice into nursing and health policy.

Nurse coaches possess the capacities necessary as change agents to bring knowledge, competencies, skills, and vision to transform their practice settings. They have a spirit of collaboration and willingness to take risks and actions toward change. Nurse coaches strive to model leadership and engage with other ethically aligned colleagues that contribute to healthy people living on a healthy planet.

TABLE 2 Crosswalk of ANA Ethics Provisions and Nurse Coach Core Values

Code of Ethics Provisions	ANA *Code of Ethics for Nurses With Interpretive Statements* and Nurse Coach Core Values	Nurse Coach Core Values
	Provision 1: The nurse practices with compassion and respect for the inherent dignity, worth, and unique attributes of every person.	
1.1	Respect for Human Dignity	Core Value 2 Core Value 5
1.2	Relationships with Patients	Core Value 2 Core Value 5
1.3	The Nature of Health	Core Value 2 Core Value 5
1.4	The Right to Self-Determination	Core Value 2
1.5	Relationships with Colleagues and Others	Core Value 2
	Provision 2. The nurse's primary commitment is to the patient, whether an individual, family, group, community, or population.	
2.1	Primacy of the Patient's Interests	Core Value 3 Core Value 5
2.2	Conflict of Interest for Nurses	Core Value 3 Core Value 5
2.3	Collaboration	Core Value 3
2.4	Professional Boundaries	Core Value 3
	Provision 3. The nurse promotes, advocates for, and protects the rights, health, and safety of the patient.	
3.1	Protection of the Rights of Privacy and Confidentiality	Core Value 5
3.2	Protection of Human Participants in Research	Core Value 5
3.3	Performance Standards and Review Mechanisms	Core Value 5

3.4	Professional Responsibility in Promoting a Culture of Safety	Core Value 5
3.5	Protection of Patient Health and Safety by Acting on Questionable Practice	Core Value 1
3.6	Patient Protection and Impaired Practice	Core Value 1
	Provision 4. The nurse has authority, accountability, and responsibility for nursing practice; makes decisions; and takes action consistent with the obligation to promote health and to provide optimal care.	
4.1	Authority, Accountability, and Responsibility	Core Value 1
4.2	Accountability for Nursing Judgments, Decisions, and Actions	Core Value 1
4.3	Responsibility for Nursing Judgments, Decisions, and Actions	Core Value 1
4.4	Assignment and Delegation of Nursing Activities or Tasks	Core Value 1
	Provision 5. The nurse owes the same duties to self as to others, including the responsibility to promote health and safety, preserve wholeness of character and integrity, maintain competence, and continue personal and professional growth.	
5.1	Duties to Self and Others	Core Value 2
5.2	Promotion of Personal Health, Safety, and Well-Being	Core Value 2 Core Value 5
5.3	Preservation of Wholeness of Character	Core Value 2
5.4	Preservation of Integrity	Core Value 2
5.5	Maintenance of Competence and Continuation of Professional Growth	Core Value 2 Core Value 5
5.6	Continuation of Personal Growth	Core Value 2
	Provision 6. The nurse, through individual and collective effort, establishes, maintains, and improves the ethical environment of the work settings and conditions of employment that are conducive to safe, quality healthcare.	
6.1	The Environment and Moral Virtue	Core Value 4

6.2	The Environment and Ethical Obligation	Core Value 4
6.3	Responsibility for the Healthcare Environment	Core Value 4
	Provision 7. The nurse, in all roles and settings, advances the profession through research and scholarly inquiry, professional standard development, and the generation of both nursing and health policy.	
7.1	Contributions Through Research and Scholarly Inquiry	Core Value 5
7.2	Contributions Through Developing, Maintaining, and Implementing Professional Practice Standards	Core Value 5
7.3	Contributions Through Nursing and Health Policy Development	Core Value 5
	Provision 8. The nurse collaborates with other health professionals and the public to protect human rights, promote health diplomacy, and reduce health disparities.	
8.1	Health is a Universal Right	Core Value 3
8.2	Collaborations for Health, Human Rights, and Health Disparity	Corc Value 3
8.3	Obligations to Advance Health and Human Rights and Reduce Disparities	Core Value 3
8.4	Collaboration for Human Rights in Complex, Extreme, or Extraordinary Practice Settings	Core Value 3
	Provision 9. The profession of nursing, collectively through its professional organizations, must articulate nursing values, maintain the integrity of the profession, and integrate principles of social justice into nursing and health policy.	
9.1	Articulation and Assertion of Values	Core Value 3
9.2	Integrity of the Profession	Core Value 3
9.3	Integrating Social Justice	Core Value 3
9.4	Social Justice in Nursing and Health Policy	Core Value 3

© 2021 Mary Elaine Southard, Barbara M. Dossey, Linda Bark & Bonney Gulino Schaub. Used with permission. Adapted from ANA, 2015a and ANA/AHNA, 2019.

Table 2 provides the following crosswalk identifying how the ANA Code of Ethics (ANA, 2015b) provisions are integrally related to the core values of nurse coaching:

Core Value 2. Nurse Coach Self-Reflection, Self-Development, and Self-Care

Self-Reflection

Self-reflection is an inner awareness of a person's thoughts, feelings, judgments, and personal values and beliefs. Adherence to the principles of nurse coaching requires a thoughtful, honest evaluation. Perception "opens the process for the intentional and conscious use of self as a therapeutic instrument in the healing process" (McElligott, 2015, p. 407; Shields, 2016). This ongoing practice reflects the commitment to the discipline to sharpen skills and correct missteps.

Reflection allows nurse coaches to decrease work fatigue and connect their critical-thinking capacities with the compassionate art of being with another (Johns, 2017; Stewart-Lord, Baillie, & Woods, 2017; Wong, 2018).

Self-Development

Self-development is a process of accepting personal responsibility for one's learning and development that involves self-reflection, self-assessment, self-evaluation, and self-care. This process invites nurse coaches to be transformational leaders and to explore many areas of their lives while noticing ways to let go of fixed ideas (Clavelle & Prado-Inzerillo, 2018), one's own suffering, and the suffering of others (Rushton, 2018). It is a discovery process of learning to embrace all experiences directly and use all the ingredients of life to move to deeper spaces of intention, presence, and healing (Schaub, 2015).

Self-Care

Self-care is the process of engaging in health-related activities that include health-promoting behaviors, feelings, and attitudes, in order to adopt a healthier lifestyle and enhance balance and well-being. Self-care occurs and changes throughout the lifespan as one uses compassion-focused awareness, reflective choices, and self-determined actions and behaviors in a meaningful way (Amaya, Melynk, & Neale, 2018; Hrabe, Melynk, & Neale, 2018; Melynk & Neale, 2018a, 2018b, 2018c, 2018d).

Self-care also includes the exploration of emotional, social, and spiritual domains. The fulfillment of self-care needs requires conscious awareness, self-responsibility, and problem-solving skills. Nurse coaches use self-care modalities as a means to refresh, renew, and re-energize so they can be a "well" of understanding, support, and presence.

Core Value 3. Nurse Coaching Process

Nurse coaches adapt nursing process terminology and interventions to coordinate person-centered care. The interventions most frequently use in the nurse coaching process are listed in Appendix D.

The Nursing Process

The nursing process involves six focal areas: Assessment, Diagnosis, Outcomes Identification, Planning, Implementation, and Evaluation. These six areas are conceptualized as bi-directional feedback loops from each component (ANA, 2015). Caring is the essence of nurse coaching practice, which honors the transpersonal dimension of the caring-healing relationship between the nurse coach and the person (Bark, 2011; Dossey, Luck, & Schaub, 2015; Rosa, Horton-Deutsch, & Watson, 2019).

Nurse Coaching Process

Nurse coaches use the nursing process with a shift in terminology and meaning to understand and incorporate the individual's subjective experience. The six areas of the nursing process transpose to the following six-step nurse coaching process (Hess et al., 2013):

1. Establishing relationship and identifying readiness for change (Assessment),

2. Identifying opportunities, issues, and concerns (Diagnosis),

3. Establishing person-centered goals (Outcomes Identification),

4. Creating the structure of the coaching interaction (Planning),

5. Empowering and motivating the individual to reach goals (Implementation), and

6. Assisting the individual to determine the extent to which goals were achieved (Evaluation).

The nurse coach understands that growth and improved health, wholeness, and well-being are the result of an ongoing journey that is ever expanding.

1. **Establishing Relationship and Identifying Readiness for Change (Assessment):**

   The nurse coach begins by becoming fully present with self and the individual before initiating the coaching interaction. Cultivating and establishing a relationship with the healthcare consumer is a priority for effective nurse coaching, and this is a relationship-centered caring process. Assessment involves identifying the person's strengths, what one wants to change, and assisting the person to determine their available resources and readiness for change. Assessment is dynamic and ongoing.

2. Identifying Opportunities, Issues, and Concerns (Diagnosis):

The nurse coach, in partnership with the person, identifies opportunities and issues related to growth, overall health, wholeness, and well-being. Opportunities for celebrating well-being are explored. The nurse coach acknowledges the individual's strengths that promote and reinforce the person's previous successes and serve to enhance further achievements. There is no attempt or need to assign labels or to establish a diagnosis when coaching. Instead, the nurse coach is open to multiple interpretations of an unfolding interaction.

3. Establishing Person-Centered Goals (Outcomes Identification):

The nurse coach employs an overall approach to each coaching interaction that is designed to facilitate achievement of the person's goals and desired results. The individual sets the agenda for the coaching session and goal achievement.

4. Creating the Structure of the Coaching Interaction (Planning):

The nurse coach may structure the coaching interaction with a coaching agreement that identifies specific parameters of the coaching relationship, including responsibilities and action plans for both the nurse coach and the individual.

5. Empowering and Motivating the Individual to Reach Goals (Implementation):

The nurse coach employs effective communication skills such as deep listening, powerful questioning, and direct feedback as key components of the coaching interaction. In partnership with the individual, the nurse coach facilitates learning and results by co-creating awareness, designing actions, setting goals, planning, and addressing progress and accountability. The nurse coach skillfully chooses interventions based on the person's statements and actions, and interacts with intention and curiosity in a manner that assists the individual toward achievement of desired goals. The nurse coach effectively uses nursing knowledge, in addition to a variety of skills acquired through coach training.

6. Assisting the Individual to Determine the Extent to Which Goals Were Achieved (Evaluation):

The nurse coach is aware that evaluation of coaching (the nursing intervention) is done primarily by the individual and is based on the person's perception of success and achievement of the person's desired goals. The nurse coach partners with the individual to evaluate progress toward goals.

Core Value 4. Nurse Coach Communication, Therapeutic Relationships, Healing Environments, and Cultural Care

Nurse Coach Communication

Nurse coach communication is a free flowing interchange of verbal and nonverbal information between and among individuals, nature, and all living beings. Nurse coaches convey empathy by carefully observing an individual to better understand their response to their illness. Viewing the individual's emotions objectively, the nurse coach has the capacity to recognize and ask questions using respectful inquiry. Empathy is the beginning of an effective therapeutic alliance. Nurse coaches are aware of strengthening individuals' self-efficacy and the personal belief that each person has the capacity to begin and sustain change toward desired behaviors (Bark, 2011; Schaub, 2015). They also focus on individuals' self-esteem, the belief that one has value and self-worth.

Nurse coaches are skilled at asking open-ended questions in which there is no simple yes or no response (Bark, 2011). Open-ended questions encourage reflection and meaningful responses. As nurse coaches listen to individuals' stories, they are careful not to lapse into pity that may be an expression of sorrow for suffering (Dossey, 2015c). Pity implies judgment and is often expressed with words or acts of comfort such as tears and a desire to spare the other from their discomfort. However, nurse coaches do convey sympathy that is feeling the sorrow or suffering of another.

Nurses, who spend more time with patients than do their physician colleagues and other clinical counterparts, carry a particularly heavy communication burden. Successful communication in nursing practice requires skill, sensitivity, and intuition. To optimize health outcomes, the nurse coach and healthcare consumer relationship relies as much on the following three aspects of coaching communication as it does on clinical observation and assessment:

- development of trust and respect;
- the understanding of and appreciation for the individual's values, perspectives, perceptions, and culture; and
- the display of empathy (Southard, 2018).

Nurse coaches engage with individuals about health and well-being by listening for and mobilizing "change talk" (Southard, 2017). These are a person's expressions that indicate intent to change or follow through with a desired goal; this change talk can be subtle and culturally specific. Nurse coaches are also attuned to listening for a person's expressions of ambivalence that may communicate a state of being indecisive or feeling two or more ways about something. Ambivalence can occur when personal values are not aligned with desired change or reveal a lack of commitment to change.

Nurse coaches use person-centered methods for motivating change by exploring and resolving ambivalence within the individual. The nurse coaching process assists individuals to communicate ideas related to decisional balance, which is the process of evaluating the pros and cons of changing or not changing (Davis, 2015a). In this communication process, nurse coaches also listen for a person's discrepancy that conveys a lack of agreement or inconsistency on steps with a decision or action steps toward healthier behaviors (Davis, 2015a). They listen for the person's communication about motivation that provides insight about what drives a person to make choices and take action (Booth, 2015). They recognize that a person can sustain change when they identify their intrinsic motivators, such as wanting to change a health behavior.

Nurse coaches use strategies that originate in compassion, the opposite of violence. This assumes that all humans have the same needs and that their actions are a means of meeting those needs (Davis, 2015b). Without compassion for another's needs and active listening, there is much that is "lost in translation." Nurse coaches are alert to signs of a person's resistance that may be heard through comments or expressions of "push back" related to change, health behaviors, or other factors. Non-verbal expressions of communication such as the use of visual cues of body language or voice inflections are also indicative of energetic information.

Therapeutic Relationships

Within the therapeutic relationship, nurse coaches recognize that each person's uniqueness and individuality is always emerging. It is through the discovery process and rediscovery that hunches, intuition, and new insights are allowed to emerge (Southard, Bark, & Hess, 2016). This opens to a right relationship that is "a process of connection among or between parts of the whole person that increases energy, coherence, and creativity" in the individual's body–mind–spirit–culture–environment (Quinn, 2016, p. 101).

Nurse coaches enter into the therapeutic relationship, listening for nuances of how the patient's story unfolds. This is the "meaning making" that is placed within the context and situation(s) that are arising in the person's life (Schaub, 2015a). From this emerges the person's potential to become more aware and to make choices that reflect personal values and beliefs toward their health, which is embodied in the nurse coaching process. As the nurse coach and healthcare consumer's relationship evolves, it becomes a co-created lived experience, with a new sense of meaning through insights that lead to healthy life choices, new possibilities and experiences, ways to form healthier relationships, and much more (Leihr & Smith, 2018).

Nurse coaches also develop respect within their individual and interprofessional relationships. Respect is not about liking someone, condoning the decisions or behaviors of others, or avoiding conflict (Rushton, 2018). Respecting individuals, colleagues, or others because they are human beings is different from respecting them for what they know or for their title or position. Demonstrating respect becomes very challenging when nurse coaches find themselves in situations where there are values conflicts or when there is no agreement with the decisions of others, or when the personality of the individual is offensive. This is extremely important in nurse coaching when a healthcare consumer makes decisions that the nurse coach does not endorse. This requires deep listening to what the individual is saying and honoring their role as the expert. The nurse coach does not aim to convince a person of a particular way of thinking or what choices they should make.

Healing Environments

Nurse coaches create a habitat for healing in their nurse coaching practices that "provides a context of caring, for the purpose of healing, which may include curing" (Quinn, 2016, p. 101). They define the environment as everything, both the external and internal factors, that surround an individual or group of people and include physical, mental, social, cultural, and spiritual dimensions. It also includes animate and inanimate objects and the climate, including seen and unseen vibrations, frequencies, and energy patterns (Luck, 2015b).

The internal environment is vital to optimal healing, and this includes how thoughts, emotions, and spirit have a direct impact on creating a therapeutic presence and a sacred space. Healing intention is to be open to the unknowing and the highest good for oneself or another. Within the healing environment, nurse coaches pay close attention to the social and environmental determinants of health.

Environmental ethics is also addressed, which is a division of philosophy concerned with valuing the environment, primarily as it relates to humankind, and secondarily, as it relates to other creatures and to the planet (*Nightingale Declaration for a Healthy World,* n.d.) A nurse coach focuses on how to have a healthier environment. For example, they may coach individuals, with permission, or respond to patient's questions on how to increase their awareness about such topics as toxic factors in their food, clothes, homes, offices, cars, communities, relationships, and much more.

Nurse coaches are environmental advocates and inform healthcare consumers about the precautionary principle when an activity raises threats of harm to human health or the environments; precautionary measures should be taken even if cause-and-effect relationships have not been fully established scientifically (Luck, 2016). Of note is that Florence Nightingale observed and used the precautionary principle and wrote in *Notes on Nursing*, "If you think a patient is being poisoned by a copper kettle, cut off all possible connection to avoid further injury; it has actually been made a question of medical ethics, what should a medical man do who suspects poison?" (Nightingale, 1860, p. 70).

In today's hospital environment, all healthcare workers face new environmental challenges and potential toxicity. Nurse coaches help increase the awareness of environmental co-factors and link information about exposures, risks, consequences, and how to make healthier choices. The preface of Nightingale's *Notes on Hospitals* begins as follows: "It may be a strange principle to enunciate as the very first requirement in a hospital that it should do the sick no harm. It is quite necessary nevertheless to lay down such a principle, because the actual mortality in hospitals, especially in those of large crowded cities, is very much higher than any calculations founded on the mortality of the same class of patient treated out of hospitals would lead us to expect" (Nightingale, 1863, Preface p. 1). Nurse coaches are alert to environmental factors that influence health. They work with interdisciplinary teams to determine if environmental exposures are adversely affecting health.

Cultural Care

Nurse coaches are challenged to deepen their understanding of cultural perspectives in health and healing. Nurse coaches are uniquely positioned to explore the soul and roots of cultural meaning that binds people, families, and communities together. They view culture as integrative, integral, and holistic while embracing a social phenomenon that weaves the past, present, and future (Engebretson, 2016). Nurse coaches recognize that culture is embedded in all individuals and groups, and it shapes experiences through a unique set of values, patterns of behaviors, traditions and rituals, and ways of seeing the world (Rosa, 2018).

As nurse coaches listen to an individual's stories, they recognize that ideas about health are deeply held and embedded in one's earliest experience, culture, and traditions. As all societies develop strategies and systems to maintain health and treat illness, honoring the familial heritage is important (Leininger, 2006). Nurse coaches not only explore how health is viewed but also consider the balance in the inner and outer worlds—natural, familial, communal, and metaphysical. These shared dimensions of culture transcend all cultures and can describe beliefs and practices used to maintain health and well-being that include food, movement, social connections, rituals, healing practices, and traditions (Luck & Dossey, 2015).

Nurse coaches view culture as the shared values, beliefs, attitudes, customs, rituals, symbols, and social structures that provide meaning and significance to an individual's or a group's human behaviors living in the world (Engebretson, 2016). In their practices, nurse coaches use cultural assessments to assist recognizing and honoring an individual's or group's cultural values, beliefs, customs, and traditions that assist with implementation of culturally congruent care.

Nurse coaches explore cultural awareness through deliberate self-examination and in-depth exploration of one's biases, stereotypes, prejudices, assumptions, and "isms" held about individuals and groups who are different (Engebretson, 2016). They are aware of individualized cultural care and are sensitive to cultural factors that influence the health and illness behaviors of an individual, family, community, and population.

Nurse coaches increase their cultural competence as they focus on the ability to interact effectively with people of different cultures and socioeconomic backgrounds, particularly in the context of human resources (Rosa, 2018). They are alert to the person's cultural history that is the process where a person is aligned with one's native culture, which can influence their capacity to change and achieve desired lifestyle goals. They encourage individuals to engage in their cultural rituals and to enact cultural beliefs and values. Rituals are healing when they include the repetition and patterns of behaviors and beliefs that have personal, healing worth (Ray, 2016).

Nurse coaches engage in healing presence and listen to individuals' stories with full intention to hear the cultural threads of their experiences (Luck & Dossey, 2015). In nurse coaching sessions, this allows the person to seek wholeness and balance, while often in the midst of vulnerability, transformation, and transition. During this deep listening process, the nurse coach shifts into mindful awareness and consciousness of co-participating with the individual's story in the healing process. Nurse coaches recognize that when listening to the person's story with present moment awareness, they become part of the person's environment. This is the healing moment of entering into an energy space or a field of shared consciousness (Dossey, 2015c). Throughout time, cultural models have held a worldview that there is body–mind–spirit–cultural–environmental interconnectedness.

Core Value 5. Nurse Coach Education and Research

Nurse Coach Education

In preparing future nurses with nurse coaching knowledge and skills, nurse coach educators are also teaching life skills so that students can be productive individuals. Nurse coach education is best done by discovery learning when developing coursework related to nurse coaching (Davis, 2015c). Within a course, a positive learning experience is created where there is trust and a safe environment. Nurse coaches establish an environment in which the students and teacher(s) are present to each other so that the teacher becomes the facilitator of holding the space. It is recommended that rituals be incorporated into the teaching such as centering at the beginning of class with a reflective practice. This sets the tone for honoring and respecting both the space between participants and the space within the classroom or workshop.

In nurse coach education, time is spent on how to shift mindset from "fixing" to "being" in addition to asking curious questions of the learner (Davis, 2015c). The nurse coaching process is a step-by-step method, with emphasis on new ways of thinking, listening, and becoming curious. In the classroom, coaching principles are applied. This includes allowing for pauses so that students have space to reflect on concepts, ideas, feelings, and experiences. This is how profound, deep learning can take place.

Nurse coach faculty encourage students to share only what they wish to share and to be honored if they wish not to share. When they choose not to share, their silence is honored (Davis, 2015c). They are encouraged to reflect on what lies beneath the silence; shame, grief, insecurity, doubt, or uncertainty, unlocking the barrier to greater clarity and direction.

Nurse coaching education should be designed to not only build on what is known but also to foster confidence, which is optimal for deep learning (Davis, 2015c). Sample coursework should include course descriptions, objectives, topics, activities, and other assignments. Engagement in group process work allows for new insights and approaches to seek solutions to real problems.

The practice of student-to-student coaching is often the first step in actualizing the theory and skills that have been learned in the classroom or online training. As progress is made in practice, students take this experience into the community for service learning. This is teaching that combines academic content with civic responsibility in a community project (Jordan, 2013). This learning is structured and supervised and enables the student to reflect on what has taken place.

Nurse Coach Research

Nurse coaches engage in a spirit of inquiry that facilitates a culture of evidence-informed and evidence-based practice and research (Taylor & McElligott, 2015). Nurse coaches are informed by and work from a diverse field of relevant research. It is important that nurse coaches continue to conduct new research recognizing that this is an essential component of the work. Nurse coaches also collaborate with interprofessional research teams to strengthen the recognition and value of nurse coaching in the broad range of clinical and community settings where they practice (McElligot et al., 2018).

Another aspect of the researcher role is that nurse coaches continually develop strong information literacy skills to effectively locate and utilize high-quality resources. Research findings are one of many possible sources of information for an evidence-based nurse coaching practice. These findings provide an important cornerstone to nurse coaching practice.

Nurse coaches contribute to research by asking researchable questions and partnering with other nurse coaches and interprofessional colleagues and researchers to design and implement research studies. A major focus includes studies that contribute to health and wellness outcomes data from practice experiences, and participating in analyzing data for future research initiatives. Future directions in nurse coaching research will push the boundaries of current methodologies that may be barriers to understanding complex and often immeasurable phenomena.

The Where of Professional Nurse Coaching: Settings for Practice

Professional nurse coaches work in all areas of nursing practice and interact with individuals, groups, families, and communities and populations (Ross et al., 2018) (see Table 3; Descriptive Characteristics of Certified Nurse Coaches). They are staff nurses, ambulatory care nurses, case managers, advanced practice registered nurses, nursing faculty, nurse researchers, educators, administrators, and/or nurse entrepreneurs in private practice, among others. They may practice in a specialty area, including but not limited to, diabetes education, cardiac rehabilitation, or end-of-life care.

Nurse coaches may focus on health and wellness coaching, executive coaching, faculty development coaching, managerial coaching, business coaching, or life coaching. The extent to which registered nurses engage in the nurse coach role is dependent on coach-specific education, training, experience, position, and the population they serve.

Table 3. Descriptive Characteristics of Certified Nurse Coaches

Primary Position	Total (n=164)	%
Nurse coach	38	23.2%
Staff nurse	37	22.6%
Nurse manager/leadership	20	12.2%
Educator (school/university setting)	13	7.9%
Nurse practitioner	13	7.9%
Case manager	13	7.9%
Clinical nurse specialist	8	4.9%
Staff development/educator	8	4.9%
Other	14	8.5%
Primary Place of Employment		
Private practice	42	25.6%
Hospital	40	24.4%
Ambulatory clinic/office	31	18.9%
School of Nursing	12	7.3%
Government/community agency	10	6.1%
Business/industry	8	4.9%
Home health agency	7	4.3%
Insurance company	5	3%
Other school setting	6	3.7%
Hospice	3	1.8%

(Ross et al., 2018) Used with Permission.

The Relevance of Nurse Coaching

Nurses fundamentally can be a catalyst in the ever evolving journey of patient-centered care. Whether working in teams coordinating care or one on one coaching, nurses can lead by example using coaching skills, attitudes, and behaviors. Measureable, data-informed improvement can be achieved when patients see scalable solutions. Nurse coaching is a consumer-driven healthcare service that contributes to positive healthcare outcomes.

Nurse Coaches in Clinical Settings

Nurse coaching is integrated into various clinical settings. While the setting may vary, the need for listening and communication skills is paramount and remains invaluable in improving patients' satisfaction both in their care and potential outcomes. In a qualitative systemic review, Newell and Jordan (2015) point to studies that indicate improved health outcomes when patients feel listened to by their providers and are actively participating in their own health-care decisions. However, the potential benefit of "patient-centered care" and "partnering with consumers (i.e., patients)" is offset by a gap in the actual communication practices of nurses who remain primarily "task-orientated" (Wellard, Lillibridge, Beanland, & Lewis, 2003).

Newell and Jordan (2015) also indicate that healthcare organizations have a lack of recognition and support for patient-centered communication, and many do not promote a culture in which the nurse could practice in this manner. Improved communication is a valuable opportunity that is being lost in terms of better health outcomes, quality of care, and patient satisfaction in the organization. This is a strong endorsement for the need to have all nurses skilled in nurse coaching.

The framework for healthcare delivery and interventions has changed dramatically over the years. Innovative approaches to providing care are warranted for seamless transitions. Complex care that had been previously delivered in the acute care setting is now provided in alternate settings. Comprehensive management and inclusion of other members of the healthcare team now enable chronically ill and vulnerable populations to remain in their homes. An example is the integration of health coaching with home pulmonary rehabilitation (Benzo et al., 2018). Home-based pulmonary rehabilitation highlights the importance of social support, and the nurse coach is a vital component that helps the patient better understand their illness, triggers, and barriers to high-level functioning.

Nurse Coaching in Education

Use of a coaching model in school nursing is a positive approach to empower students and encourage healthy choices at an early age. For many, school nurses have an advantage of following students over time. This enables tailoring coaching interventions based on developmental milestones and a deep understanding of the student's needs and goals. Wellness centers YMCAs, YWCAs, and fitness centers are other places that nurse coaches can provide services to enhance the ability of the organization to assist with transformation for their members.

Nurse Coaching in Private Practice

Nurse coaches in private practice enjoy the benefits of "being their own boss," creating a flexible work schedule, selecting their target market and niche, and often working from home. The entrepreneurial model requires business acumen and marketing strategies for success.

Additional venues for nurse coaching are working with people who have chronic conditions such as diabetes, congestive heart failure, cardiovascular disease, and more. Extending nurse coaching—from health promotion and disease prevention to chronic care and advanced illness—broadens the practice and establishes the function of nurse coaching across all areas of care.

Some nurse patient advocates and nurse navigators find that coaching skills are invaluable as they work with colleagues, families, and individual clients. Nurse coaches may want to work with certain populations like nurses new to the profession, or new mothers who are finding their way as parents. Coaching those who are experiencing high levels of stress, either personally or professionally, is very rewarding. Needless to say, these clients are so thankful for coaching services because they are usually in a very difficult situation without many resources or support. The nurse coach walks with them as they rebuild their lives, and uses the experience gained over the years with other clients to see opportunities for change.

Nurse coaches can also combine coaching with specific private practice services such as energy work, massage, advocacy, or cannabis nursing. Nurse coaches who practice energy and bodywork have reported that combining these interventions can help clients set clearer healing intentions, increase motivation and experience more lasting positive changes.

As medical cannabis is becoming more prevalent within states, nurses working in this area may find coaching certification or training to be beneficial. Coaching helps clients better understand resources and options as they find new levels of comfort and healing.

Nurse Coaches Working in Communities and Groups

Many people are becoming aware of the fact that they can make choices and take actions that will help them to maintain and improve their health. An example of this growing awareness and interest in self-improvement was evidenced when a board-certified nurse coach offered a program on health and wellness through a school district, teaching a series of evening classes for the community. The nurse was delighted when the class rapidly filled up with eager participants. Through meditation, breathing, and imagery practices, they learned to be aware of inner thoughts and obstacles and recognize that healthy choices were possible. The program was very successful and became a place of support and community connection. Participants requested to have the group offered repeatedly. Some of the participants asked the nurse coach to work with them privately during the times the school-based program was not available. It is clear that this sense of connection was of significant value to the nurse coach.

Loneliness and isolation have been recognized as a major global public health problem, particularly for elderly people with minimal social networks (Aoki et al., 2018; Cacioppo & Cacioppo, 2018). Loneliness has been recognized as a condition that causes irritability, depression, self-centeredness, and a 26% increase in premature death. Loneliness has also been identified as a risk factor for dementia (Sutin, Stephan, Luchetti, & Terracciano, 2018). Addressing social determinants of health becomes a factor not just in the elderly population but across the lifespan of individuals. Nurse coaches can make an impact in diverse settings, such as libraries, faith communities, and senior centers, in order to meet the individual where they are at. Using group dynamic coaching skills, the nurse coach can provide services face to face, telephonically, in video conferencing or in small groups.

Group Health Coaching

Group health coaching offered by nurse coaches is a cost-effective approach for providing care. Group health coaching was recognized as an important next step in making health promotion available to greater numbers of people (Armstrong et al., 2013). One of the key benefits of this coaching model was the creation of a "sense of community." It also promotes a greater sense of commitment and follow-through. The grouping of healthcare consumers with the same medical challenge has been recognized as beneficial peer support. Examples include landmark programs such as Dean Ornish's (1990) work with heart disease patients and Kabat-Zinn's (1991) work with pain patients, as well as the support groups that are offered for other physical challenges. These programs speak to the value of people coming together for support in creating and sustaining healthful choices.

Nurse coaches in private practice find that group coaching is a way to provide affordable care to more healthcare consumers. For example, women's health is an area that lends itself readily to the value of nurse coaching groups. Fitness, Yoga, or T'ai Chi teachers bring their nurse coaching skills to healthcare consumers wanting the benefit of group support. This support can be a means for participants to maintain motivation and connect with a greater sense of purpose. Nurse coaches who work as school nurses have been able to offer groups to parents, teaching meditation and other stress management skills for their own self-care as well as for their children.

Faith-Based Communities

Nurse coaches are also skilled and ready to bring health and wellness support to a wide range of faith-based communities. In many instances, parish nurses are the community's primary contact with healthcare. Public health and mental health nurses have collaborated with parish nurses by teaching nurse coaching skills. Adapting and individualizing stress management programs and self-care practices for the faith-based population reflects the fundamental aspect of mind–body–spirit–culture and environment components of health, wellness, and well-being. Another example of this is a nurse coach who is providing self-care and stress management groups for grief support groups or those that have experienced loss through separation or divorce.

Community Health Programs

The Brookings Institute (2016), as part of an initiative titled *Building Healthy Neighborhoods Series,* included a report titled "Nurses as Intermediaries in the Promotion of Community Health: Exploring Their Roles and Challenges." This report referenced the Institute of Medicine's (IOM, 2017) statement that underscored the critical importance of nursing in adequately addressing public health. The report emphasized that an effective healthcare system "needs to coordinate medical facilities with the behavioral and economic drivers in communities that are most related to long-term health." The report acknowledged that nurses are the essential intermediaries in this process because of their broad range of specialties and diversity of roles and work settings (Butler & Diaz, 2017). As clinical nurse leaders (CNLs), and as consultants and practitioners in community centers, schools, parishes, and other settings, nursing's presence pervades our culture. The report stated that nurses, in comparison to other healthcare providers, are trained more as "system thinkers" with a holistic perspective of healthcare consumers and "have intimate insight into the patient experience." It also emphasized that nurses, as well as being highly trained in their clinical knowledge, can be skilled in leadership and care coordination. This presents an opportunity for nurses skilled in executive coaching and team management coaching skills to be leaders in building systems for the promotion of community health (McNally & Cunningham, 2010).

An example of a nurse coach-led, community-based program, and its potential and challenges, was studied in China (Huang et al., 2017). Nurse coaches were connected with a patient population of high-risk coronary heart disease individuals. The purpose was to detect and manage individuals at significant risk for coronary heart disease (CHD). They were recruited from two communities and followed for 6 months. There were 120 participants in the program. They all were tested for systolic blood pressure (SBP), health-related quality of life (HRQoL), and self-rated depression scale (SDS). Sixty participants in the control group received the usual care, which included a brochure about CHD prevention and a health consultation. The other treatment group of 60 received a health consultation and group education sessions, which were two lectures a month for the first 3 months, followed by at-home and telephone coaching support for 3 months.

The outcomes demonstrated a significant positive effect for the clients receiving the education and coaching interventions. The SBP of the treatment group decreased, and there was no change in the SBP of the usual care group. The depression scores of all the participants had indicated mild depression. Following the intervention, the treatment group had a significant reduction in SDS scores from initial baseline to post intervention. The HRQoLs of both groups were similar prior to onset of treatment. At completion, both groups had improved HRQoL, but the intervention group's improvement was significant, and the usual care group's improvement was not. Summarization of the conclusion of the study was that the nurse-led, community-based education and nurse coaching intervention in a CHD high-risk population showed positive effects on SBP, HRQoL, and SDS. While the specific details of the training and implementation of nurse coaching is not clearly delineated in this study, it strongly shows the value of nurse coaching interventions as a primary prevention strategy in community health systems.

Transforming Unhealthy Work Environments

Workplace Violence and Incivility

Workplace violence and incivility is widespread in healthcare professions (Ahmad, Al Ramawi, Masadeh, & Atoum, 2015). This violence has been identified as "violent acts, including physical assaults and threats of assault, directed towards persons at work or on duty" (OSHA, n.d.). This problem includes verbal violence such as threats, hostility, and harassment. These actions come primarily from patients, but also from family members and visitors. Violence among colleagues, referred to as "horizontal violence . . . includes bullying, screaming, constant criticism, eye-rolling, denigrating talk, sabotage, and ignoring someone" (Schablon, Wendeler, Kozak, Nienhaus, & Steinke, 2018).

These incidents are vastly underreported, especially bullying and other forms of verbal abuse that occur in hospitals, clinics, nursing homes, and other settings (OSHA, 2015). Nurses are recipients of this violence at higher rates than other healthcare professionals (OSHA, 2015). The International Council of Nurses in 2009 stated that workplace violence directed toward nurses occurs in healthcare settings worldwide, and subsequent to these events, nurses often suffer physically and/or emotionally, experiencing stress, depression, and sleep disorders. These traumatic events also impact the other nurses and staff (Ahmad Al-Rimawi, Masadeh, & Atoum, 2015; Martinez, 2016), and can be the impetus for nurses leaving their profession or developing significant anxiety when working in particular settings (Edwards, M. & Blackwood, K.M., 2017).

In Finland, a major cross-sectional survey compared the association between patient aggression and the well-being of nurses working in psychiatric and non-psychiatric settings. The factors measured regarding well-being included self-rate health, sleep disturbances, psychological distress, and perceived work ability (Pekurinen et al., 2017). The study was created to look at factors contributing to the serious nursing shortage that was anticipated to occur in the coming years. The total population consisted of 5,288 nurses, with 923 nurses working in a psychiatric setting, 4,070 working in medical and surgical settings, and 295 in emergency settings (Pekurinen et al., 2017).

The study demonstrated that although psychiatric nurses faced patient aggression more often, their well-being was better, and they had less sleep problems compared to medical and surgical nurses. The researchers concluded that psychiatric nurses were more likely to recognize a disturbance of their psychological well-being resulting from the aggression and to seek help for this.

The research about the negative effect of violence and incivility on nurses also cites the negative influences on colleagues, patients, and the healthcare system. There is significant underreporting of these events. Some of the reasons for this have been cited as a sense of responsibility for the event, fears of being blamed, or lacking the therapeutic communication skills to feel safe discussing the event. It is important for nurse managers and leaders to create an environment where nurses feel safe to report what they have experienced and receive the emotional support they need (Schablon et al., 2018).

Using Coaching Principles to Create a Healthy Culture

In recognition of the need for optimal healing environments, it would be of great value if nurse managers and leaders had professional nurse coaches on staff to work with other members of the healthcare team. Skilled nurse coaches can provide an environment that is open and safe for nurses to pause and be focused on their own well-being. Equally as impactful would be having nurse managers or staff nurses trained in nurse coaching skills. In a recent study with nurse managers, it was shown that coaching skills enhanced transformational leadership of their teams of nurses. It also resulted in improved team management and cohesiveness that resulted in better quality of patient care (Westcott, 2016).

Both the American Organization for Nursing Leadership (AONL, formerly known as American Organization of Nurse Executives) and National Center for Healthcare Leadership (NCHL) have challenged nursing leaders to implement the coaching approach in their work with teams. The introduction of coaching is a catalyst for bringing the best forward in all members of a team. Creation of a coaching culture is valued as a creative process that is open to the effective, accountable, and cohesive action plans applicable in many contexts (McNally & Cunningham, 2010).

Support for Healthy Work Environments

Nurses face many challenges in today's healthcare culture. In acute care medical settings where they are continually caring for severely ill and dying patients, nurses are experiencing compassion fatigue (CF) and secondary traumatic stress (STS). These vulnerabilities must be addressed early on to ensure that neither the nurse nor the patient is adversely affected (Upton, 2018). Nurses with greater emotional vulnerability and experiencing CF have also become susceptible to substance use and misuse (Jarrad, Hammad, Shawashi, & Mahmoud, 2018). In a recent study, emotional exhaustion was seen as the primary reason for RNs and licensed practical nurses (LPNs) working in an acute care setting to leave their jobs (Havaei, MacPhee, & Dahinten, 2016).

A national survey of certified nurse coaches was conducted to examine the value of this role for advanced practice registered nurses (Ross et al., 2018). The study focused on work settings and health conditions and addressed motivating factors of nurses pursuing nurse coach board certification. It also indicated how coaching was of personal value as well as a benefit for the people they were coaching. The nurses worked with a wide range of individuals who had different medical conditions. The primary condition addressed was anxiety and stress with cardio-metabolic conditions and pain. When asked why the nurses chose to pursue coach certification, they expressed the intention to deepen their ability to alleviate the pain and suffering that they witnessed in their clinical work. The value of coach training was seen as improving their interpersonal relationships, healthy behaviors, and increased job satisfaction. There was also an interest in bringing nurse coaching into a private practice. The nurse practitioners valued the credential of being board certified as a nurse coach in strengthening the validity of their work. The researchers concluded that advanced practice registered nurses could gain ground in the ongoing battle to improve the health of the nation by adding nurse coaching skills into their practice (Ross et al., 2018).

High-Performing Interprofessional Teams

Professional nurse coaching practice facilitates relational coordination, interprofessional meetings, and healthy team environments by having a positive impact on healthcare processes and outcomes. Interprofessional collaborative practice (IPCP) as defined by the World Health Organization (WHO, 2009) is "when multiple workers from different professional backgrounds work together with patients, families, caregivers, and communities to deliver the highest quality of care" (p. 7). "Relational coordination" is the mutually reinforcing process of communicating and relating for task integration and a powerful driver of performance when work is interdependent, uncertain, and time constrained.

Care that is high quality and supported by the dimensions of shared goals, shared knowledge, and mutual respect can lead to better healthcare outcomes. Integral to the process of work that constitutes nurse coaching practice are the theoretical constructs of both nursing and social sciences.

Nurse coaching is implemented and translated through high-quality relationships and frequent, high-quality communication. The mutual influence and understanding of these constructs are essential to engage in problem-solving communication, rather than shaming or blaming to attain better healthcare outcomes.

The evidence to support best practice-based interventions that build interprofessional collaboration still needs further research. Bringing the nurse coach skill set into interprofessional team coaching is an area for further exploration. Team coaching has been utilized to improve healthcare delivery systems by increasing interprofessional collaboration (Godfrey, Andersson-Gare, Nelson, Nilsson, & Ahlstrom, 2014). Godfrey et al. (2014) studied an interprofessional team, working in intensive care nurseries. Paired teams of nurses and physicians as well as other groups received coaching and were also trained in coaching. There were paired teams of nurses and physicians as well as other groups. Four areas of focus proved to be crucial in the effectiveness of the coaching:

1) *context*—understanding the current conditions of the work site,

2) *relationships*—establishing trust and rapport between the team coach and staff,

3) *helping*—learning specific communication skills plus support and guidance to facilitate interprofessional cooperation, and

4) *technical*—materials and resources to continue the staff goal of greater collaboration.

The implications for nursing management addressed the value of team coaching in building and strengthening workplace relationships.

The use of a structured interprofessional team coaching model would offer encouragement to keep participants energized and improve the quality of healthcare. In nurse coaching, this can be developed as an area of advanced practice.

Current Landscape of Nurse Coaching Education

The current trends in nurse coaching education continue to evolve as more programs develop and become incorporated into academic settings. The baccalaureate level for nursing as an entry level to the profession is needed for the professional nurse coach to meet the needs of global health issues within the context of a culturally diverse and aging population. Planning and implementing nurse coaching curriculum relevant to 21st century healthcare issues and clinical practice requirements includes incorporation of teaching preventive health behavior, outreach to high-risk clients, reducing environmental hazards, and providing culturally appropriate care.

Independent Certificate and Academic Nurse Coach Programs

The following are examples of nurse coach program requirements.

Independent Certificate Programs

In the United States, nurses can select from a variety of nurse coach educational programs. When considering a program, there are important questions to ask:

- What is your professional philosophy and how can the program meet your future professional needs?
- What is the basic philosophy (e.g., holistic, functional, allopathic) of the educational program?
- Who is their target market? (e.g., only nurses, other licensed professionals)
- What are faculty areas of practice?
- Does the program meet requirements for AHNCC certification?
- How long does the program take to complete?
- How/when is the program offered? (e.g., format-online, face-to-face, hybrid, residential)
- How much does the program cost? and how long has it been offered?
- Are Continuing Education hours offered?

Independent nurse coach programs offer their own *certificate*, which is a "branded" certificate that verifies completion of the program.

Academic Programs

Course work in nurse coaching is becoming embedded in baccalaureate level, graduate, and advanced practice registered nurse (APRN) programs across the country. Studies have supported and concluded that coaching is a valuable strategy for APRN practice and a valuable benefit for patient engagement (Hayes, 2007; Ross et al., 2018). Academic certificate programs need to be vetted with similar questions as those listed for independent certificate programs.

Nurses not yet trained as nurse coaches often say they are already coaches. Many nurses also say, "We are all holistic." The term "coach" is defined in Merriam Webster's dictionary (n.d.) as "someone who is a private tutor, one who instructs, trains, and especially one who instructs players in the fundamentals of a sport and directs team strategy." Based on the common understanding of the word, one might agree with those nurses. However, the meaning of the term "coach" has expanded over the past decades.

The same can be said of the term "holistic." Merely educating healthcare consumers on how to improve and modify their lifestyles often proves ineffective. For years, professionals have been providing patients with educational pamphlets on healthy behavior and the adverse effects of poor health habits. Holistic nurses embrace a philosophy focused on unity, wellness, and the unique relationship of self, others, and the environment. Healing the whole person requires a pivotal contrast, orientation, worldview, and focus.

The monumental paradigm shift for nurses is the realization that nurse coaching is not about just providing the education but also supporting and helping the individual understand their health challenges in a broader context. Allowing the healthcare consumer to be the expert takes practice, and a true shift in consciousness, with the underlying skill of understanding behavior change. This is such a tremendous change from what nurses have been taught—to move into a place of beginner yet have the courage to ask the powerful questions that spark inquiry.

Nurse coaches realize they can help people so much more by partnering with them rather than setting the educational agenda for them. For example, one bedside nurse coach, who worked on an orthopedic unit, started asking her patients what they wanted to do in the upcoming summer. Her patients responded with stories about wanting to go on vacation or to keep up with young grandchildren. After becoming clear on their intrinsic motivation, the patients acted differently: they asked to get up, were ready for PT early, worked hard, and were discharged sooner. The nurse coach's colleagues noticed these changes and asked what she was doing. When she told them, they were baffled by how one question made such a difference. The change came from more than just one question; it was a different way of interacting with her patients.

Nurse coaching does not take more time, effort, or additional work. Instead, it decreases stress for both parties involved and brings a sense of accomplishment. The coaching approach is also a powerful tool for nurse leaders and executives. The skills of active listening, negotiation, and asking powerful questions can be an important complement to achieving success as a nurse leader.

Working in this way, nurse coaches see progress—of individuals, groups, and within organizations. Many nurses comment after completing coaching coursework, that they had not been practicing nurse coaching accurately in the past. They learn to integrate and reconfigure how to "be with" a patient using a new skill—making them more effective and feeling more productive.

Board Certification for Nurse Coaching

The American Holistic Nurses Credentialing Corporation (AHNCC) has administered the national certification examination in nurse coaching since January 2013. This Magnet-recognized and nationally accredited examination is based on the professional nurse coach competencies and Role Delineation Study (AHNCC, 2017). More information about Nurse Coaching board certification can be found at www.ahncc.org. The AHNCC Nurse Coach board certification requirements are as follows:

- Unrestricted, current U.S. RN license.
- A minimum of a baccalaureate (BS, BSN) degree in nursing from an accredited academic institution (international candidates must have their baccalaureate nursing degree evaluated to determine that their program is equivalent to a U.S. baccalaureate nursing degree program).
- Active practice as an RN for a minimum of 2 years full time or 4,000 hours part time within the past 5 years.
- Completion of a minimum of continuing nursing education (60 CNE) contact hours, accrued over the past 3 years, that include content consistent with the nurse coach core values and nurse coach competencies.
- Sixty hours coaching experience that has been mentored and/or supervised by a certified nurse coach supervisor, and a validation letter from a board-certified nurse coach.

Entry into Beginning Nurse Coach Practice

The current entry level for nurse coach practice (see requirements above) is two years of active practice as an RN along with a baccalaureate degree. Nurse coaching is relationship-centered and relationship-based and furthers these dynamics by allowing and extending opportunities for personal and professional growth.

Registered nurses who have completed graduate course majors outside of nursing may become a nurse coach.

Academic and Continuing Education

The academic and continuing education trajectory for competency development related to coaching may include coursework in refining coaching skills, appreciative inquiry, motivational interviewing, or specialized domains such as nutrition. Advanced practice registered nurses become forerunners in the health coaching movement, caring for medically complex, at-risk populations both within healthcare organizations and in private practice. With a growing emphasis on health promotion and disease prevention, advanced practice registered nurse coaches address wellness interventions, chronic conditions, and genomic implications for risk.

Advanced practice registered nurse coaches negotiate on individual, unit, and institutional levels to intervene, empower, and improve interpersonal relationships, health behaviors, and organizational culture. As change agents, they build bridges across traditional healthcare practices to develop personalized approaches to maximize health and well-being for individuals at all stages of life across diverse populations and settings.

Being able to address the whole person during coaching sessions, rather than a targeted individual concern under time limitations, requires a trust-building context in which shared decision-making occurs. In claiming the future of the advanced practice registered nurse coach, the expertise, innovation, and leadership skills of APRNs will be called upon to guide and shape practice and policies. Developing research agendas, identifying novel scientific questions, encouraging new thinking, and exploring unanswered questions will guide advanced practice registered nurse coaches' evidence-based practice. Appendix H provides emerging competencies for the graduate and the advanced practice registered nurse coach. Continuing education (CE) coursework related to coaching can vary and be used for recertification as well as professional development. While personal enrichment courses are helpful, they are not reflected or used for recertification.

Professional Competence in Nurse Coaching

Clinical competence is one of the significant merits of nursing, and its evaluation can lead to recognition of fields requiring improvement (Sherwood & Barnsteiner, 2017). Along the educational continuum, students advance and demonstrate basic knowledge and learning outcomes. Theoretical knowledge along with an identified framework are observed in clinical environments and evaluated for proficiency. The constant evaluation of clinical competency is carried out by third parties (i.e., organizational policy managers and peer reviewers). For Nurse Coaches, the continued commitment to personal mastery and their own growth and development include an evaluation of a new skillset for professional development and quality assurance. Areas of self-reflection encompass occupational and organizational tasks, practice, environment, critical thinking, and therapeutic interventions. This self-evaluation of clinical competence helps Nurse Coaches pay attention to and improve their own clinical functions through raising their self-awareness and commitment to change.

In general, very few studies have been conducted on the clinical competence condition of nurses (Watson et al., 2017). While Nurse Coaches engage in supervision of coaching skills once a coaching program has been completed, being able to improve skills can raise the quality of services given to healthcare consumers. Thorough planning, reflecting, evaluation, and documentation is necessary. Self-assessment assists nurses to maintain and improve their practice by identifying their strengths and areas that may need to be further developed (Meretoja et al., 2004).

In addition, the process of analyzing and tracking information about one's coaching interventions will add to the knowledge, attitudes, and skills toward expert practice. Structured note taking, in this area is an important caveat to coincide with clinical assessment (establishing relationship and identifying readiness to change), planning (individual goals), and implementation (interventions), but also for continual evaluation (outcomes) and quality improvement (self-reflection).

Professional Trends and Issues

Health and Healthcare in the United States

Understanding potential trajectories in health and drivers of health is crucial to guiding long-term investments and policy implementation (Foreman et al., 2018). The future is not predicted to provide corrections to the downward trend. Globally, most independent drivers of health were forecast to improve by 2040, but 36 were forecast to worsen (Foreman et al., 2018). Life expectancy in the United States (78.6 years) has decreased slightly over the past 2 years and is expected to remain at lower levels, while globally life expectancy is forecasted to increase by 4.4 years (Murphy, Jiaquan, Kochanek, & Arias, 2018). Since 1990, body mass index (BMI) has continued to rise in almost all countries, with this trend continuing to increase at least until 2040 (Foreman et al., 2018). A high BMI is linked to chronic disease (Kearns, Dee, Fitzgerald, Doherty & Perry, 2014).

The one bright spot in the U.S. health overview is in the area of infant mortality: the U.S. rate is lower globally but is still higher than many developed countries (Foreman et al., 2018). Unfortunately, the advantage of infant health seems to be overcome by declining health as children age and become adults. More than 117 million Americans, almost half the adult population, live with at least one chronic disease (CDC, 2016). Less than 23% of American adults met the recommended amount of physical activity needed to promote health and wellness (Blackwell & Clarke, 2018), and only 1 in 10 Americans eat the daily recommended amount of fruits and vegetables (Lee-Kwan, Moore, Blanck, Harris, & Galuska, 2017). In addition to diet and exercise, smoking and high alcohol consumption also factor in when considering mortality and morbidity (Rail, 2016). Furthermore, from 2016 to 2017, the suicide rate in the United States increased by 3.7% (CDC, 2018).

Research is beginning to evaluate how nurse coaches help clients reduce and reverse chronic conditions. This approach of facilitating healthy lifestyle behavior change leads to higher levels of well-being. Adult clients with chronic conditions such as multiple sclerosis, cancer, pain, depression, and substance use disorder described their lived experience of being coached by nurse coaches (Delaney, Bark, & Barrere, 2019). The clients ranged in age from 28 to 78 years old and had been receiving coaching for durations of 4 months up to 8 years. Eight themes emerged as they reported their coaching experiences:

- They entered coaching seeking guidance to navigate life's challenges.
- Coaching felt like a safe, sacred place.
- They felt empowered and accountable.
- They developed strategies to access different ways of knowing.
- They found answers within themselves.
- They made healthy behavioral changes.
- They formed a new caring relationship with themselves.
- They created a brand new approach to life.

As already mentioned in the Preamble of this book, our healthcare system is not addressing the needs of people due to lack of engagement, disempowered healthcare consumers, overprescribing, medical errors, and lack of continuity and coordination of care (Petri, et al., 2017; WHO, 2009; Gusovsky, 2016; Makary & Daniel, 2016; Jowsey et al., 2016). When healthcare consumers are empowered and supported by nurse coaches, they can address complex issues by finding reasonable treatment that matches their values, along with proper medications, which are warranted and make sense to them. Nurse coaches can support, advocate, educate, and provide resources when individuals ask them to perform that role. The nurse coach can also be the one that helps bridge the gap, supporting a safe transition from one level of care to the next (Delaney & Bark 2019).

Creating a Sustainable Nurse Coach Workforce

A nursing shortage in the United States is predicted for the future. Limited faculty, difficulty in finding clinical practice settings, nurse burnout, a large number of Baby Boomer nurses retiring, and fewer people entering the nursing profession are all factors that lead to this trend (Haddad & Toney-Butler, 2018).

The nurse coaching workforce numbers may differ from the overall shortage for several reasons. First, older nurses who are planning or about to retire will be leaving hospital systems, but some may still want to stay connected to nursing and so traverse into the role of nurse coach. These nurses describe a desire to utilize their years of knowledge and proficiency in helping people, because they are not ready to fully leave the profession. Sometimes the need to augment their retirement savings is a factor.

Many envision nurse coaching as an encore career in which they could begin a private practice or work part time for an employer while having the opportunity to co-create one-on-one, person-centered partnerships, which is what called them into nursing in the first place. Many describe past positions where they lost that ability to feel like they had time to pursue a healing relationship with patients. They see nurse coaching as a way to provide meaningful interaction, perhaps the freedom to work from home through telecoaching, and the ability to be more in control of their time. Some Baby Boomer nurses who have experience in leadership and management envision a nurse coaching practice where they can coach those who are still in the healthcare system, offering them a relationship that draws on their years of experience and wisdom.

Second, some younger and middle-aged nurses have sound reasons to pursue nurse coach certification. They may want to avoid burnout and leave the high-pressure working environment of many healthcare systems. The thought of working in a less stressful setting with individuals who want to change and become healthier is inviting, interesting, and rewarding. They may want to create more work-life balance and see nurse coaching as a way to meet that goal.

Another reason for the popularity of nurse coaching is that all ages are showing a growing interest in wellness and health promotion. Millennial nurses (born 1981–1996) encompass the largest number of nurses in the current workforce, and they are more interested in professional development than the earlier generations of nurses (Bell, 2013). Nurse coaching is one way that they can enhance their skills and practice.

Bridging all generations of the nursing workforce, job satisfaction, and personal growth are two other reasons for the growing proliferation of nurses interested in nurse coaching. Several studies indicate that nurse coaching offers increased job satisfaction regardless of previous position or place of employment. Retention and recruitment are factors of interest for all employers since it costs 40–65% of an annual salary to replace an employee (Dube, Freeman, & Reich, 2010; Kantor, 2017). Ross et al. (2018) also report that certified nurse coaches find personal development and improved relationships in all areas of their life as well as experiencing higher levels of health.

Another trend in healthcare that affects nurse coaching has to do with collaboration, new partners, and a move to local and home-based care that is changing healthcare across the United States. For example, on November 2018, CVS acquired Aetna for a cost of $69 billion dollars (Cassel, 2018). The CVS president and CEO stated:

> *By delivering the combined capabilities of our two leading organizations, we will transform the consumer health experience and build healthier communities through a new innovative health care model that is local, easier to use, less expensive, and puts consumers at the center of their care.* (CVS Press Release, 2017)

CVS, as well as other retail pharmacies, are already employing coaches in their setting, so as mergers continue to unfold, this could be a perfect place for nurse coaches to work with individuals who have complex health conditions and medication adherence challenges.

The shift to bringing healthcare to individuals at a local level also fits with the Healthy People 2030 vision, mission, plan of action, and overarching goals for a healthier nation (Office of Disease Prevention and Health Promotion, 2018). Some services are moving into the community, but others have moved into the home, for example, assisting with "rite of passage" for birthing and dying. Recently, a new service being delivered in the home is an innovative program pertaining to substance use disorder. Instead of sending the addicted person to a spa-like setting to learn new behavior patterns, this program brings the team to the home, and the education and treatment occur around the kitchen table or in the living room with the whole family and system. In this way, the whole system is healed, and relapse is greatly reduced. The program uses nurse coaches and a coaching culture.

Nurse Coaching Across State Lines

State nurse practice acts (NPAs) statutes, codes, and regulations are managed by the state boards of nursing. Although there is some common ground in NPAs, there is much variation. As compact state agreements progress, there have also been many advances in telemedicine and telecoaching. Thus, nurse coaches are required to follow their state NPA, regulations, and guidelines. They do not practice across state lines unless they have an Enhanced Nurse Licensure Compact (eNLC) license that allows for coaching healthcare consumers in other compact states (Nurse Licensure Compact, 2015; Ghani, 2019).

Nurse coaches need a nursing license for the states in which their clients reside if it is different from their own residence of professional practice. When nurse coaches work for companies that have clients in different states, the nurse coaches will need additional licenses for the states in which their clients reside. Since this can be costly and cumbersome for nurse coaches to have nursing licenses in several states, the efforts to build the compact state coalition speaks to the need for flexibility in this field (Brown, 2018; Fathi, Modin, & Scott, 2017; Ghani, 2019). Currently, there are 34 states in the compact agreement, and more are pending inclusion (NCSBN, 2017).

Reimbursement for Nurse Coaching Services

As of the revision of this document in October 2020, there is no insurance or government reimbursement for nurse coaching. However, nurse coaching sessions or services can be allocated to a Flexible Spending Account (FSA) by using a National Provider Identification (NPI) number. Nurse coaches, like all healthcare professionals, can apply for an NPI number from the Centers for Medicare and Medicaid Services (CMS). Healthcare professionals need to follow the requirements and policies closely or they may be required to pay back funds collected for services they have provided or incur penalties. Emerging Category III codes are in the process of being beta tested.

Additional avenues for nurse coaching reimbursement need to be created. Nurse coaches and advocates of nurse coaching, such as schools and certifying organizations, should join forces to lobby for nurse coach reimbursement in Congress and in the CMS.

Opportunities to work as a Nurse Coach vary. Healthcare systems and insurance companies, as well as corporations, hire nurse coaches to work with their members. If the nurse coach is in a private practice, the majority follow a fee-for-service model.

Today, much of healthcare is viewed from the lens of the managed-care industry where value-driven care performance measures such as the Healthcare Effectiveness Data and Information Set (HEDIS®) are used as a benchmark. The measures are developed and maintained by the National Committee on

Quality Care (NCQA, 2020). HEDIS® was designed to allow consumers to compare health plan performance to other plans, to collect information on the performance of physicians, and to track individual year-to-year performance. HEDIS® includes more than 90 measures across six domains of care. The six domains of care are:

1. Effectiveness of Care

2. Access/Availability of Care

3. Experience of Care

4. Utilization and Relative Resource Use

5. Health Plan Descriptive Information

6. Measures Collected Using Electronic Clinical Data Systems

These data are collected through surveys, medical chart audits, and insurance claims for hospitalizations, medical office visits, and procedures. Many health insurance companies hire nurse coaches to provide services for Medicare enrollees based on adherence to HEDIS® guidelines. The distinct difference between current nurse coaching practice and this rigorous process of following performance measures is that the setting of goals in coaching is patient driven rather than plan determined. While HEDIS® measures focus on processes of care and provider "buy-in," nurse coaching focuses on individual "buy-in" while promoting healthy behaviors.

Striving to meet the benchmark goals and constraints for condition-specific measures can, for some patients, be perceived as an unachievable goal and a deterrent for intrinsic motivation. As a quality improvement review, nurse coaches are at the intersection of practitioners and healthcare consumers and can effectively assist individuals to balance meeting the benchmarks with their own healthcare goals, while understanding their own barriers and resistance to modify behavior.

The Distinction Between Nurse Coaches and Non-Nurse Coaches

Nurse Coaches have a breadth and depth of experience together with knowledge of health and the healthcare system that is not commonly held by other healthcare practitioners or those in the fitness and wellness field. Nurses work with individuals and groups experiencing acute and chronic illness often based on poor lifestyle choices. They understand the complexity of decision-making and treatment plans they often encounter. Below are some of the specific reasons that professional nurse coaches are hired by individuals and companies instead of other health and wellness coaches.

Nurse coaches:

- Address the whole person from a holistic/integral perspective following the holistic nurse principle standards and competencies;
- Understand their scope of practice avoiding the legal risk of diagnosing, prescribing, or treating individuals. Litigation is costly at many levels;
- Use evidence-based or evidence-informed interventions;
- Understand when to refer to other resources;
- Are knowledgeable about transitions of care and how to communicate those levels;
- Have more than basic healthcare knowledge and can alert individuals to critical health situations;
- Often have years of experience in the healthcare setting and can help individuals navigate a difficult, confusing, and sometimes frustrating system;
- Stay attuned to a wide variety of healthcare information sources;
- Easily switch to consulting or providing education when requested by the healthcare consumer;
- Follow the trend of home or community-based services;
- Advocate for an individual; and
- Model "walking the talk" and exemplify what helps both them and healthcare consumers to greater well-being and health.

A salient point is that nurses are trusted by the public and were chosen again as the profession whom the public trusts the most. They feel that nurses are honest and ethical (Gallup, 2020).

Nurse Coaching, Leadership, and Organizational Culture

A significant trend in the coaching industry is using coaching to build talent and leadership. The difference between a good leader and a great leader is that the latter not only completes projects well but also does so in a way that inspires long-term motivation and sustainable results within the team. Organizations are finding that:

Coaching is both a mindset and a set of behaviors by which leaders enable their people to assess an issue, identify appropriate actions, participate in decision making, and achieve positive business results while simultaneously helping them learn and contribute. Leaders who are good coaches inspire and challenge others in their organizations to grow and develop; ultimately, such leaders are capable of achieving stronger business results than those less supportive and collaborative. (Accenture. com, 2019)

A coach leader will use coaching competencies to promote trust within the group; use and facilitate the effective communication skills of deep listening, powerful questions, and direct communication; and watch for a shift in behaviors while supporting accountability and learning (McCarthy, Feuerlicht, Ohn, & Silverstone, 2018).

This trend has not been ignored by nursing leadership. McNally and Cunningham (2010) are very clear about the value of coaching when they say that ". . . those leaders who have worked with a professional coach and then learned how to coach others are clearly more effective in creating cultures of accountability and orchestrating action on many fronts" (p. 54). They continue to assert that there is still limited empirical evidence on its benefits to nurse managers.

In the past, the work of providing leadership development and coaching was reserved for professional coaching and organization development practitioners. Now leaders at all levels are being asked to use the coaching approach with team members. Both the American Organization of Nurse Executives and the National Center for Healthcare Leadership directly and indirectly identify coaching as an essential component of executive practicing. Integrating coaching into your leadership practice extends your reach and impact. (McNally & Cunningham, 2010, p. 7)

Nurse coaches are not only using their coaching skills to correct specific performance concerns with employees and to facilitate success in their teams, but some are also using coaching principles to create healthy organizational cultures. An organizational culture is "how things are done" in a particular unit, group, or company. Sometimes cultures are not consciously created or addressed, and "how things are done" create a toxic environment with devastating consequences. People may think it is acceptable to complain, gossip, say unkind things about others, bully an imbalanced coworker, or make fun of an underperforming coworker.

Workplace violence and incivility is the result of such a culture. This type of culture thrives on a lack of empathy, poor communication skills, and emotional imbalance within the organization. Building a sustainable coaching culture aids organizations in creating the next generation of leaders—it is one way by which a company can execute leadership development at scale. For an organization to cultivate a coaching culture, it must focus on principles, perspectives, and behaviors. In an environment where people are treated with respect and trust, feel part of a community, have positive relationships, receive feedback they can do their work well, feel empowered, have fun, and feel creative. Then they can be productive, have pride in what they do, learn both personally and professionally. When they are fairly compensated for their work, are rewarded for company growth, and have the tools and space they need to do their jobs well, they are motivated. Healthy cultures produce increased productivity, low staff turnover rates, and profitable operations as well as grow future leaders. (Bark, 2001; Cable & Graham, 2018; Hawkins, 2012; McCarthy et al., 2018). Establishing healthy cultures and authentic leadership based on nurse coaching does not happen by accident. It requires concerted effort, time, and resources to create specific programs and training for effective leadership. Such programs nurture coach champions who will bring the approach to all levels of practice and service (Bark, 2001; Hawkins, 2012; McCarthy et al., 2018). This is being done in some settings, investing in creating coaching skills at all levels of the organization by:

- Making sure coaching should be a central part of any leadership development curriculum, with a learning approach that emphasizes action learning and simulated interactions;

- Providing ongoing support and development for leaders in modeling coaching behaviors, and then, for individuals at all levels to adopt those behaviors; and

- Measuring, recognizing, and rewarding effective coaching as it is demonstrated by individuals and teams across the organization to create stronger accountability and celebrate when significant achievements are made.

Research in Nurse Coaching

A literature search on over 40 years of nurse coaching practice has elicited varying results related to evidence-based best practice in nurse coaching (See Appendix I). Many of the studies that are identified describe nurses who do coaching. Few studies describe the type or quantity of the coaching, nor do they specify the coach training of the nurses. The training may vary from a 1-hour in-service program on motivational interviewing techniques to a 60-hour course required for nurse coach certification. Looking at outcomes from these studies with such limited information can be misleading.

Cognizant of the need for better research about nurse coaching, academic centers, institutional organizations, and government agencies are producing meaningful studies. Research that merits attention and adds credibility to nurse coaching has addressed the efficacy of outcomes, the impact of training on the nurse coaches, themselves, and the role and application of nurse coaching in various settings.

A systematic review of health and wellness coaches conducted by Wolever et al. (2013) was pivotal in health and wellness coaching literature. The review revealed that nurses contributed to the majority of articles on health and wellness coaching from all categories of medical and allied health professionals. Nurses also contributed 40.1% to research and practice articles and 51% to conceptual articles (Wolever et al., 2013). In addition, nurse coaching warranted attention from the National Institute of Health by sponsoring a study of certified nurse coaches in advanced practice (Ross et al., 2018; See Appendix I).

Documentation of Nurse Coach Practice

Today's healthcare landscape requires data management, analysis of outcomes, the ability to retrieve the work, and also the expertise to describe individual and population-based needs. Mainstream application requires the field to coalesce enough in language and concept to be consistently understood by implementers, health systems, researchers, policymakers, purchasers, and of course, patients themselves (Peek, 2013). Unifying a field with consistently understood concepts and definitions can be extremely useful in an emerging field such as nurse coaching.

An example of using standardized terminology to document nursing practice is the use of the Omaha System. The Omaha System (www.omahasystem.org; Martin, 2009) is a research-based, comprehensive practice and documentation standardized taxonomy designed to describe client care. It is based on rigorous and extensive research and enables collection, aggregation, and analysis of clinical data worldwide.

The Omaha System consists of client problems or nursing diagnoses referred to as the Problem Classification Scheme. Nursing interventions with associated categories and targets are referred to as the Intervention Scheme. Outcomes measurement scales for client knowledge, behavior, and status (KBS) are referred to as the Problem Rating Scale for Outcomes. Healthcare leaders are using the Omaha System as a tool to address meaningful goals; monitor and enhance care quality, efficiency, and value; engage patients and families; improve care coordination; and promote population health.

Originally used in public health settings, the Omaha System was designed to be relatively simple, computer-compatible, and used by interdisciplinary practitioners to document and communicate information. It is also consistent with nurse coaching based on a holistic foundation reflecting a partnership with practitioners and the value of a problem-solving process (Martin, 2015).

Having a standardized method for charting nurse coaching services and interventions offers a solid foundation to study nurse coaching practice. Standardized terminology can show how coaching can inform organizational culture and enhance nurse coaching practice, education, research, and policy. A meaningful study that has taken this need even further identified the feasibility of using the Omaha System as a framework for documentation of nurse coach practice (Southard et al., 2016). The three aims of the study were to:

- Evaluate content validity of nurse coach case studies;
- Test accuracy of nurse coach graduates identifying Omaha System terms for nurse coach interventions; and
- Explore the feasibility of analyzing nurse coach case study data.

For the purpose of this study, surveys were emailed to 400 graduates of two nurse coach education programs. Nurse coaches self-reported little to no experience using standardized terminologies for documentation prior to completing the survey questionnaire.

Across the three case studies, 95.7% of nurse coaches agreed that the case studies were realistic, and 89.3% agreed that they would use similar interventions. Nurse coaches accurately identified Omaha System interventions for the case studies 84.3% of the time. In addition, the feasibility of analyzing nurse coach practice data was demonstrated through use of case study data in aggregate (Southard et al., 2017).

The Omaha System should be considered for development of a standardized, evidence-based guideline for nurse coaching practice. Standardized terminology can direct the way nurses use coaching skills and can be a framework for reflection for how the practitioner thinks about what to do next. The use of this tool can provide nurse coaches with a "thinking shortcut" to aid in successfully engaging individuals or communities and to ultimately validate sustainable healthcare outcomes. The impact of data accessibility and translation of value-based interventions can help to change healthcare by moving the concept of coaching into everyday clinical practice.

More case studies need to be mapped to the Omaha System, along with comparative effectiveness trials of different types of interventions. Many nurses enrolling in DNP or PhD programs are interested in focusing their research on nurse coach interventions, which will augment evidence-based practice. Further, developing measures such as the Omaha System techniques and using technology for information management will determine a cost-benefit analysis of nurse coaching interventions.

In particular, nurse coaches in private practice need to adhere to documentation guidelines for privacy, security, and accuracy. An open-source electronic health record (EHR) can be an invaluable tool to capture coaching interventions and follow trends for client progress. Appendix G is an example of an open-source EHR.

Remote Monitoring and Coaching

Nurse coaches commonly work in the wellness and behavior change arena, which has seen an upsurge of health apps, online offerings, and home monitoring devices. Platforms have been created to link patients, providers, medical institutions, and consultants using wearable or Internet-connected devices and sensors. This offers timely data analysis and the opportunity for care coordination and collaborative health planning and intervention.

Depending on the individual, the benefit of this integration can far exceed the cost of the equipment or device. Many of the external devices are meant to help increase motivation. However, for some individuals, the external reminders may alter the objective by contributing to anxiety or obsessive behaviors. Used in conjunction with nurse coaching support, these products can be an invaluable asset in increasing intrinsic motivation and contributing to goal achievement.

Telehealth Trends

Due to the increasing pervasiveness of chronic diseases and rising healthcare costs, the American telehealth market is expected to extend to $16.8 billion by 2020 (Masterson, 2018). Healthcare costs in the United States have risen every year since 1960, and in the past 20 years, these costs have exploded, increasing by 261% through 2016 (Haudenschield & Blachek, 2018).

As of 2016, there were 72 telehealth bills in legislation; eight have been enacted, eight have failed (NCSB, 2016). According to the Center for Medicare and Medicaid Services (CMS), in 2016, there were 17 million people under Medicare. Expanding the use of telehealth strategies for Medicare beneficiaries with chronic conditions asks the question of whether telehealth can help to improve quality, reduce costs, and increase care coordination for beneficiaries with chronic conditions. As background, Medicare has historically provided limited coverage for telehealth services. Before authorizing payment for telehealth-delivered services, Medicare usually requires that providers, technology (mainly live video), and patient locations need to be in certain types of healthcare facilities or in rural areas. CMS, in their rule, expresses concern that these requirements may be limiting the coding for new kinds of services that utilize communication technology.

Implications of Telehealth for Nurses and Nurse Coaches

According to the National Council on State Boards of Nursing (NCSBN, 2016), state boards do not provide specific guidance regarding telehealth. Licensure is based on the location of the individual patient, so the provider needs to be licensed in the state where their patient resides.

The distinction needs to be made regarding telehealth monitoring and telehealth nurse coaching. *Telehealth monitoring* consists of providing wound assessment at a distance, monitoring vital signs such as blood pressure, blood glucose levels, heart rate, or weight via devices for self-measurement, or monitoring movements in and around the home via activity monitors. The services trigger alarms for nurse case managers to intervene and assess based on organizational protocols. *Telehealth nurse coaching* can be provided via telephone or video conferencing platforms in compliance with privacy and confidentiality rules.

Nurse practitioners (APRN) are eligible for reimbursement in the areas of Interprofessional Internet Consultation (CPT codes 99452, 99451, 99446, 99447, 99448, and 99449) (Bindman, 2013). These codes would cover interprofessional consultations performed via communications technology such as telephone or Internet (Malerba, Richman, Koziak, & Radler, 2018). This would support team-based approaches to care that are often facilitated by EHR technology. Nurse coaching, combined with technology, supports goal setting, health tracking, and resolving barriers (Fazio et al., 2019). Fazio and colleagues (2019) conducted research using surveys and documentation from motivational interview-based coaching sessions between study nurses and intervention participants. Of the 132 cases reviewed, types of success predominantly fell into five categories:

1) change in health behaviors;

2) change in mindset or awareness;

3) change in engagement with healthcare resources;

4) change in physical or emotional health and;

5) change in health indicators.

Important changes in individuals' health and well-being may be overlooked or undervalued if providers strictly follow only biomarkers.

Nurse coaches need education and training to bring technology and coaching together. Nurse coaching telehealth practices require the knowledge, skills, and attitudes to execute professional nurse coaching activities using this platform. Subcategories include general, technological, clinical, health promotion, communication, and implementation skills. Knowledge of ethical, legal, and regulatory considerations is an important component in telehealth nurse coaching. Communication skills, coaching skills, the ability to combine clinical experience with telehealth, clinical knowledge, ethical awareness, and a supportive attitude were seen as the most important competencies for nurses who provide telehealth (van Houwelingen, Moerman, Ettema, Kort, & ten Cate, 2016).

The nurse coach's knowledge, self-efficacy, and listening skills are key competencies when engaging individuals using telehealth services. As video conferencing becomes more utilized for health coaching, the regulations for protection of privacy need to be clearly followed. These services would require strict adherence to legal, licensure, and documentation parameters.

Healthy People 2030

On January 2019, the U.S. Department of Health and Human Services (HHS) solicited public comments on the proposed framework for Healthy People 2030 (Office of Disease Prevention and Health Promotion, 2018). Included in the Healthy People 2030 proposal are the vision, mission, foundational principles, plan of action, and overarching goals for a healthier nation. A challenge for Healthy People 2030 is to guide the United States in achieving our population's full potential for health and well-being so that we are second to none among developed countries. The plan for Healthy People 2030 is to set national goals and measurable objectives to guide evidence-based policies, programs, and other actions to improve health and well-being. It seeks to facilitate the development and availability of affordable means of health promotion, disease prevention, and treatment.

Future objectives for Healthy People 2030 need to include nurse coaches, since they provide specific strategies and interventions to promote and sustain health in a more comprehensive manner for partnering with clients. As nurse coaching develops as a reliable approach to shared decision-making and patient-centered care, validation of interventions and analysis of core strategies will be needed.

Nurse coaching represents key opportunities to support the Healthy People 2030 initiative and to advance research for evidence-based interventions in areas where evidence is needed.

Population Focus: Generational Trends and Future Wellness Behavior

Although making generalizations about groups of people can oversimplify an individual's unique values, needs, characteristics, and behaviors, nurse coaches realize that looking at generational characteristics can offer some guidelines to further inquire and possibly augment nurse coaching practice. Significant differences among generations as it relates to healthcare expectations and preferences have been identified below.

The Baby Boomer generation (1944–1964) is so called because, prior to the Millennial generation, they were the largest group of people born in the United States. Baby Boomers numbered 74 million in the last census (Fry, 2018). This subset of the population tends to lead more sedentary lives, has high sugar intake, and suffers from chronic disease. Baby Boomers prefer face-to-face communication with healthcare practitioners and personal relationships. A goal of staying young and vital can drive them to look at lifestyle issues. Even though they did not grow up in an IT world, they use and value it for information (Sandle, 2017; Cangelosi, 2020). Baby Boomers can be attracted to nurse coaching because it is a relational-based interaction built on trust and authenticity. Connecting with the services of a nurse coach can assist them in building healthy lifestyle habits for life.

The Gen X generation (1965–1979) can be characterized as being diverse, balanced risk-takers, self-reliant, and pragmatic. They tend to be skeptical and often shop for healthcare and services as if they were purchasing a retail item. Those from the later years of Gen-X were raised on instant gratification, independent thinking, inner creativity, and addiction to change (Sandle, 2017; Cangelosi, 2020; Newman et al., 2017). They expect to be allies in a healthcare situation and encourage partnerships with their providers. Looking for a third opinion is par for the course. They are often the decision-makers for the generations above and below them, so they impact healthcare to a great degree (Fronstin, 2018). Key to nurse coaching is shared power, which those of Gen X appreciate. Encouraging people to look at a variety of options is part of coaching, so this cohort is a good fit for nurse coaching.

The Millennial generation (1981–1996) makes up the largest generation since the Baby Boomers (Fry, 2018). They have technology skills and tools, and in general, would rather use the Internet to address a health issue than go to a doctor. Many want healthcare to be convenient and low cost. Often they incorporate proactive wellness approaches into their lifestyle. They may be more open to telehealth options for concerns (Sandle, 2017; Cangelosi, 2020).

Telehealth and nurse coaching are a good fit for the Millennials since it can be very convenient and lower in cost than other interventions.

The Gen Z generation (1995–2015) is the newest generation to be named. Health and medical concerns are usually under the control of their parents, but from studies on this new generation, they are predicted to be less trustful of "big pharma" and healthcare systems as they grow older (Newman et al., 2017). The research also indicates that sales of wearable monitoring devices are high with this group (Newman et al., 2017). As we look ahead, those in Gen Z seem well positioned to accept a new innovative wave of healthcare. Scientific concepts and practices based on disease interception will be common, people will know their DNA mapping, and cancer might be a disease of the past (Sandle, 2017; Newman et al., 2017). Designing products and services for this generation takes insight into the teenage world, which some companies can find challenging (Forbes et al., 2018). Those in Gen Z may be more open to prevention as well as holistic, integrative, or integral approaches to health and well-being. It will be interesting to watch how Gen Z responds to nurse coaching as they age and have more control over healthcare choices.

Each generation exhibits characteristics of distinctive ethics, values, and healthcare needs. Nurse coaches consider all these characteristics and wellness requirements within their practice. Savvy consumers are now seeking clinical and nonclinical wellness providers. Improving care and dialogue with each generation requires nurse coaches who understand and articulate these perspectives and environments.

Nurse Coaching and Healthcare Policy

Opioid-related mortality has reached epidemic levels in certain rural areas of the U.S., such as Appalachia, New England, and the Mountain West, while remaining relatively low in others, such as the Delta South and Great Plains. Explanations for geographic variation in opioid mortality are unclear, contributing to ineffective policies and interventions (Rigg, Monnat, & Chavez, 2018).

In order to shape legislation, research is needed on current best practices to address policy. As an example, ensuring care providers deliver nondrug, non-opioid treatment for pain is a new campaign from the Integrative Health Policy Consortium (IHPC) and partners. It recommends nonpharmacological approaches as first-line pain treatment (ihpc.org). The opioid crisis is a major concern nationally. In a recent survey, the IHPC is a unique interprofessional federation of organizations focused on health creation—the proactive promotion of and focus on prevention, wellness, and well-being.

As the policy and advocacy voice of integrative health and wellness professionals, the IHPC has achieved groundbreaking success toward the transformation of health and healthcare delivery, even as the prevailing paradigm of healthcare remains entrenched in a disease-based philosophy. This national strategy has gained momentum and needs to include nurse coaches as an integral member of the action plan and team. Nurse coaches lead change and transform care in a landscape crippled by lack of agreement on terms of health coaching criteria, prerequisites, and principles. The internally consistent framework of nursing along with the dimension of collaboration is the leverage of nurse coaching principles and practice. The complexity of healthcare requires a professional who understands both the nuances of the landscape and the challenges and intricacies of human behavior related to illness and well-being.

Summary of the Scope of Nurse Coaching

There have been many changes in nurse coaching practice since the publication of *The Art and Science of Nurse Coaching: The Provider's Guide to Scope and Competencies*, 1st edition (Hess et al., 2013). While the definition of nurse coaching has not been altered, there is expansion and more detail when identifying the "who," "what," "where," "when," and "how" nurse coaching is practiced. The tenets, core values, and holistic philosophy of nurse coaching form the foundation for the core competencies that follow the nursing process and professional responsibilities for practice.

Issues and themes highlight the burgeoning landscape of nurse coaching and look at growing pains, hopes, and opportunities. Coaching is being integrated into nursing education at all levels with consequences that will grow nurse coaching in exciting ways that we cannot even predict at this time. The call for solid research to support the efficacy of nurse coaching practice will increase credibility and expand the role. Nurse coaching continues to have the potential to help millions of healthcare consumers and will change the healthcare landscape. Empowering clients provides the opportunity for nurse coaches to experience and remember the reasons that brought them into the nursing profession, with pride and satisfaction.

Development and Function of the Competencies of Professional Nurse Coaching Practice

The Professional Nurse Coaching Scope of Practice is accompanied by the description of the Six-Step Nurse Coaching Process and the associated competencies. The Professional Nurse Coach competencies related to ANA's Standards of Professional Performance characterize a competent level of behavior in the professional role activities related to ethics, culturally congruent practice, communication, collaboration, leadership, education, evidence-based practice and research, quality of practice, professional practice evaluation, resource utilization, and environmental health. Motivational Interviewing, Appreciative Inquiry, Negotiation and Direct Communication are embedded within the competencies. In December 2020, ANA's Board of Directors affirmed these published competencies of professional nurse coaching for a term of five years.

Six-Step Nurse Coaching Process

The Six Step Nurse Coaching Process describes a competent level of Nurse Coach practice as demonstrated by the foundational model of the nursing process. Nurse coaches use the nursing process with a shift in terminology and meaning to understand and incorporate the individual's subjective experience. The six areas of the nursing process transpose to the following six-step nurse coaching process:

1. Establishing relationship and identifying readiness for change (**Assessment**)

2. Identifying opportunities, issues, and concerns (**Diagnosis**)

3. Establishing person-centered goals (**Outcomes Identification**)

4. Creating the structure of the coaching interaction (**Planning**)

5. Empowering and motivating the individual to reach goals (**Implementation**)

6. Assisting the individual to determine the extent to which goals were achieved (**Evaluation**).

Step 1. Assessment

The Nurse Coach:

▶ Becomes fully present to self and individual prior to collecting data pertinent to the coaching interaction.

▶ Co-creates a relationship between the Nurse Coach and the individual that promotes trust and intimacy.

▶ Recognizes and respects the individual as the authority on own health and well-being.

▶ Explores with the individual why coaching is being considered at this time and what they want to address during the coaching interaction.

▶ Ensures the individual, or group sets the agenda for the coaching session and holds the client's agenda throughout the session.

▶ Helps the individual assess stage of readiness for change (pre-contemplation, contemplation, preparation, action, maintenance).

▶ Incorporates various types of knowing, including intuition, and validates this intuitive knowledge with the person when appropriate.

▶ Explores, through powerful questions and feedback, multiple sources of information to assist the client to become aware of areas for coaching.

Step 2. Diagnosis

The Nurse Coach:

▶ Clarifies the client's issues and concerns and/or opportunities for change based on the whole person assessment data.

▶ Confirms the client's issues and concerns and/or opportunities with the client.

▶ Tracks the client's issues and concerns and/or opportunities in a manner that leads to identification of the client's goals that will be the focus of the coaching process.

Step 3. Outcomes Identification

The Nurse Coach:

- ▶ Involves the client in formulating goals that are specific, measurable, action-oriented, realistic, and time-lined.
- ▶ Facilitates the client's process of self-discovery related to establishment of the client's goals.
- ▶ Facilitates the client's exploration of alternative ideas and options relevant to goal-setting.
- ▶ Supports the client's inner wisdom, intuition, and innate ability for knowing what is best for self.
- ▶ Realizes that new goals will emerge as the client changes and evolves.

Step 4. Planning

The Nurse Coach:

- ▶ Assists the client to identify strategies to attain goals.
- ▶ Creates with the client an action plan with clearly defined steps and anticipated results.
- ▶ Explores with client potential obstacles to goal attainment and possible responses to these challenges.
- ▶ Adjusts plan as desired by the client.

Step 5. Implementation
Before the coaching interaction the Nurse Coach:

- ▶ Becomes fully present, centered, and grounded.
- ▶ Reviews client status and/or progress from previously obtained data.
- ▶ Minimizes distractions for self and encourages client to do the same.

At the beginning of the coaching interaction the Nurse Coach:

- ▶ Explores, with the client, an outcome for the coaching session that is achievable in the time allotted.

▶ Briefly explores progress since last coaching session, with particular attention to accomplishments, challenges, or barriers relevant to current session.

Throughout the coaching interaction the Nurse Coach:

▶ Remains fully present, centered, and grounded.

  ▶ Supports the client in directing the agenda/focus of the coaching session.

  ▶ Acknowledges client and identifies strengths for change.

  ▶ Maintains an interested, open and reflective approach to the client.

  ▶ Is comfortable with silence or pausing to assist the client with reflection and finding new understanding or next steps.

  ▶ Accesses and trusts her/his own intuition and perceptions of the client.

  ▶ Draws upon the precepts of the human energy field/system to assist client in achievement of goals.

▶ Creates a safe, supportive environment that fosters intimacy and trust.

▶ Continuously exhibits authenticity (honesty, sincerity, personal integrity).

▶ Demonstrates respect for client's subjective experiences/story, perceptions, learning style, and culture (e.g., beliefs, values, and customs).

▶ Provides ongoing support for new ideas, behaviors, and actions that may involve risk-taking and fear of failure and/or fear of success.

▶ Obtains client's consent to coach client in areas of vulnerability.

▶ Chooses what is most effective in the moment from a variety of coaching strategies and implements as appropriate.

▶ Focuses on what the client is saying and is not saying to understand the meaning in the context of the client's desires and to support the client's self-expression by employing such skills as deep listening, relevant use of language, powerful questioning, and direct communication.

  ▶ Deep Listening

- Accepts, explores, reinforces, and encourages the client's expression of perceptions, concerns, beliefs, suggestions, etc.

- Recognizes in-congruencies between body language, words used, and the tone of voice.

- Paraphrases, reiterates, and summarizes what client has said to ensure understanding and clarity.

- Focuses on the essence of the client's communication when client becomes involved in long explanatory descriptions.

- Allows the client to express strong feelings without judgment in order to facilitate movement towards achievement of goals.

- Acknowledges client's ambivalence to change and helps identify barriers.

▶ Relevant Use of Language

- Uses language, including metaphors and analogies, which assist the client to explore perspectives, uncertainties, or opportunities for change.

- Uses language that is nonjudgmental, appropriate, and respectful.

- Uses language that reflects the client's worldview, beliefs, and values.

▶ Powerful Questioning

- Asks open-ended questions that create greater insight, clarity, and/or new possibilities and learning.

- Asks questions that move the client towards desired goals.

- Asks questions that evoke discovery, insight, commitment or action (e.g., those that challenge the client's assumptions).

- Uses inquiry for greater awareness, clarity, and understanding.

▶ Direct Communication

- Provides feedback in a clear and direct manner.

- Shares insights with client in ways that are practical and meaningful.

- ▶ Explores client's assumptions and perspectives to evoke new ideas and discover new possibilities for action.

- ▶ Challenges the client to stretch and be challenged, while maintaining a comfortable pace with the client.

▶ Employs integrated, holistic communication skills including deep listening, relevant use of language, powerful questions and direct communication, allowing a client to fully explore and articulate what they are hoping to achieve through the coaching relationship.

- ▶ Supports the client's inner wisdom, intuition, and innate ability for learning.

- ▶ Identifies with the client additional areas for learning and development.

- ▶ Assists the client in uncovering underlying ambivalence, concerns, typical and fixed ways of perceiving self and the world, interpretations of experiences, and differences between thoughts, feelings and actions.

- ▶ Helps the client identify barriers to change.

- ▶ Helps the client identify strengths and opportunities for learning and growth.

- ▶ Acknowledges client resistance as an opportunity for self-awareness and growth.

- ▶ Shares information with client that inspires broader perspectives.

- ▶ Encourages and supports the client to experiment and to apply what has been learned from the coaching interaction.

- ▶ Assists the client to determine actions that will enable the client to demonstrate, practice, and deepen new learning.

- ▶ Facilitates the client in taking action that will most effectively lead to achievement of desired goals and prevent relapse.

At the end of the coaching interaction the nurse coach:

- ▶ Inquires of the client if coaching session outcomes have been achieved.

- ▶ Identifies the connection between where the client is and where she/he wishes to go.

- ▶ Identifies with the client the next specific action steps and a timeline that will lead to achievement of desired goals.

- Assists the client to manage progress by holding the client accountable for stated actions, results, and related time frames, while maintaining a positive and trusting relationship with the client.
- Determines with the client when the next coaching interaction will occur.
- Periodically, if relevant, prepares, organizes, and reviews information, including past and
- Periodically, as indicated, reviews and revises the coaching plan with the client.
- Ends the coaching interaction in an energetic, positive, and supportive manner.

5A. Coordination of Care

The Nurse Coach:

- Develops relationships with other health providers to promote cohesive, coordinated, continuity of care.
- Works with patients in making health care decisions based on the fullest understanding of information in the context of a patients values and preferences.
- Establishes and maintains a plan of care (POC), jointly created and managed by patients. The POC outlines the patient's current and long term needs and goals for care, identifies coordination needs and addresses potential gaps. The POC tracks current progress toward patient goals.
- Provide and coordinate services as needed with additional resources in the community to help support patient's health and wellness to meet their care goals.

5B. Health Teaching and Health Promotion

The Nurse Coach:

- Assesses patient health beliefs and values to better understand patient's future determined goals.
- Establishes baseline parameters to define the context of potential health teaching.
- Facilitates planning of interventions to serve as an objective basis for monitoring and evaluation.

- Designs Health Promotion interventions based on quantitative and qualitative baseline parameters.
- Applies Health Promotion interventions at the request of the patient.
- Evaluates progress made toward achievement of objectives, to determine the effectiveness of interventions and to serve as a basis for improvement on Health Promotion strategies.

Step 6. Evaluation

The Nurse Coach:

- Assists the client to evaluate effectiveness of strategies in relation to the client's responses and the attainment of the expected and unfolding goals.
- Supports client autonomy by recognizing the client is the determinant of progress and success.
- Documents evaluation of progress and attainment of coaching goals.

Competencies Associated with ANA Standards of Professional Performance

Standard 7. Ethics

The Nurse Coach:

- Integrates ethical provisions in all coaching interactions.
- Uses *The Code of Ethics for Nurses with Interpretive Statements* (ANA, 2015) to guide practice and communicate the foundation of the Professional Nurse Coaching Practice.
- Clearly communicates to the client and others the distinctions among coaching, consulting, counseling, and teaching.
- Provides coaching in a manner that recognizes and respects the client's autonomy, dignity, rights, values, and beliefs.
- Maintains an effective coaching relationship that is congruent with the coaching agreement and within the boundaries of professional nursing practice.

▶ Values all life experiences as opportunities to find personal meaning and cultivate self-awareness, self-reflection, and growth.

▶ Maintains client confidentiality within legal and regulatory parameters.

Standard 8. Culturally Congruent Practice

The Nurses Coach:

▶ Promotes culturally congruent practice for nurses, educators, and researchers.

▶ Uses application of evidence-based nurse coaching practice that is in agreement with the preferred cultural values, beliefs, worldview, and practices of the healthcare consumer and other stakeholders.

▶ Design and direct services for diverse consumers to improve access, promote positive outcomes, and reduce disparities.

▶ Create a discrimination-free healthcare environment.

▶ Demonstrates respect, equity, and empathy in actions and interactions with all healthcare consumers.

▶ Participates in lifelong learning to understand cultural preferences, worldview, choices, and decision-making processes of diverse consumers.

▶ Creates an inventory of one's own values, beliefs, and cultural heritage.

▶ Applies knowledge of variations in health beliefs, practices, and communication patterns in all nurse coaching practice activities.

▶ Identifies the stage of the consumer's acculturation and accompanying patterns of needs and engagement.

Standard 9. Communication

The Nurse Coach:

▶ Employs skillful communication in all aspects of the coaching interaction.

▶ Understands that skillful communication is a fundamental component of Professional Nurse Coaching Practice.

▶ Communicates, when requested by client, with family, significant others, caregivers, health care providers, and others to assist and enhance the client's achievement of coaching goals.

Standard 10. Collaboration

The Nurse Coach:

▶ Collaborates with others to assist clients in achieving goals.

▶ Uses effective communication and change skills with individuals and groups to collaboratively identify and achieve individual, group, and organizational goals.

▶ Works collaboratively with other health and wellness coaches in interprofessional development initiatives.

▶ Collaborates with others to promote nurse coaching as a way to enhance client outcomes.

Standard 11. Leadership

The Nurse Coach:

▶ Demonstrates leadership in the promotion of effective Nurse Coaching for clients.

▶ Advances the role of the Nurse Coach among health professional and coaching colleagues and in professional organizations.

▶ Develops cognitive, emotional, moral, and spiritual intelligence to enhance leadership skills.

▶ Promotes the success of others by using effective Nurse Coaching interventions.

▶ Demonstrates energy, excitement, and a passion for quality Nurse Coaching.

▶ Willingly accepts that mistakes will be made by self and others when taking risks to achieve goals.

▶ Displays the ability to define a clear vision, associated goals, and a plan to implement and measure progress toward goals.

Standard 12. Education

The Nurse Coach:

▶ Attains knowledge and competency that reflects current Nurse Coaching practice.

▶ Participates in ongoing educational activities to enhance the Nurse Coaching role.

▶ Documents and maintains evidence of Nurse Coaching competency.

▶ Develops and uses a broad knowledge base related to holistic/integral nursing, integrative health, health systems, professional coaching competencies, counseling, health education, health promotion, and nursing practice issues.

Standard 13. Evidence-Based Practice and Research

The Nurse Coach:

▶ Integrates evidence and research into Nurse Coaching practice

▶ Uses the best available evidence, including theories and research findings, to guide and enhance the Professional Nurse Coaching Practice.

▶ Participates with others to establish research priorities and to identify research questions or areas for inquiry related to the Professional Nurse Coaching Practice.

▶ Participates in research activities related to the Professional Nurse Coaching Practice.

Standard 14. Quality of Practice

The Nurse Coach:

▶ Systematically enhances the quality and effectiveness of Nurse Coaching practice.

▶ Participates in quality improvement to enhance the Professional Nurse Coaching Practice.

▶ Contributes to the education of others concerning the Professional Nurse Coaching Practice.

▶ Documents Nurse Coaching interactions in a responsible, accountable, and ethical manner to facilitate quality review and promotion of effective Nurse Coaching practice.

▶ Uses creativity and innovation in Nurse Coaching practice to improve client outcomes.

▶ Analyzes organizational systems for barriers to effective implementation of the Professional Nurse Coaching Practice.

▶ Advocates use of the *Professional Nurse Coaching: Defining Scope of Practice Competencies* to evaluate and enhance the quality of practice.

Standard 15. Professional Practice Evaluation

The Nurse Coach:

▶ Evaluates one's own Nurse Coaching practice in relation to professional practice standards and guidelines, relevant statutes, rules, and regulations. The Nurse Coach is engaged in ongoing personal and professional self-development.

▶ Utilizes the *Professional Nurse Coach: Scope of Practice and Competencies* to evaluate and enhance quality of practice.

▶ Considers the effect of one's personal values, culture, spiritual beliefs, experiences, biases, and education on the provision of Nurse Coaching services to individuals, groups, and organizations.

▶ Provides Nurse Coaching services in a manner that is appropriate and sensitive to culture and ethnicity.

▶ Engages in self-evaluation of coaching practice on a regular basis, identifying areas of strength as well as areas in which additional development would be beneficial.

▶ Obtains evaluative feedback regarding one's own coaching from clients, peers, and professional colleagues and takes appropriate action based upon the feedback.

▶ Pursues Nurse Coach Certification as a way to demonstrate competency and to promote the Nurse Coaching role to employers, clients, and the public.

▶ Recognizes that the Professional Nurse Coaching Practice is enhanced by ongoing self-development to promote physical, mental, emotional, social, moral, and spiritual well-being.

▶ Receives personal and professional coaching to enhance quality of Nurse Coaching practice.

▶ Integrates knowledge from research on coaching into practice.

Standard 16. Resource Utilization

The Nurse Coach:

▶ Considers factors related to safety, effectiveness, cost, and impact on practice in the planning and delivery of Nurse Coaching services.

▶ Evaluates factors such as safety, effectiveness, availability, cost and benefits, efficiencies, and impact on Nurse Coaching practice when suggesting options for the client that would result in the same expected outcome.

▶ Assists the client, as appropriate, in identifying and securing appropriate and available services to facilitate achievement of client goals.

Standard 17. Environmental Health

The Nurse Coach:

▶ Considers the impact of the internal and external environment of self and client when providing Nurse Coaching services.

▶ Understands that healthy environments encompass both internal and external environments

▶ Recognizes that individual (physical, psychological, emotional, spiritual) and cultural, social, and historical factors influence internal and external environments.

▶ Considers the internal and external healing environments of self and client regarding contribution to client goal achievement.

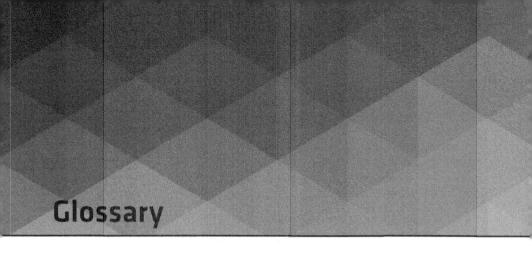

Glossary

American Association of Colleges of Nursing. The American Association of Colleges of Nursing (**AACN**) is the national voice for academic nursing. **AACN** works to establish quality standards for nursing education; assists schools in implementing those standards; influences the nursing profession to improve healthcare; and promotes public support for professional nursing education, research, and practice.

Active imagination. A process of conscious formation of images by the client as a technique or method to access deeper information and personal wisdom to facilitate changes; may include guided imagery.

Advanced Practice Registered Nurse Coach. A board-certified nurse coach who is a licensed advanced practice nurse with additional training or education in nurse coaching. An APRN is a registered nurse who has completed an accredited graduate level education program preparing her or him for the role of certified nurse practitioner, certified registered nurse anesthetist, certified nurse midwife, or clinical nurse specialist; has passed a national certification examination that measures the APRN role and population-focused competencies; maintains continued competence as evidenced by recertification; and is licensed to practice as an APRN.

Aesthetic knowing. The art of nursing that focuses on how to explore experiences and meaning in life with self or another that includes authentic presence, the nurse as a facilitator of healing, and the artfulness of a healing environment. Aesthetic knowing is the combination of knowledge, experience, instinct, and intuition that connects the nurse with a patient or client in order to explore the meaning of a situation about the human experiences of life, health, illness, and death. Aesthetic knowing calls forth resources and inner strengths from the nurse to be a facilitator in the healing process. Aesthetic knowing is the integration and expression of all the other patterns of knowing in nursing praxis.

Affirmation. An intentional declaration of a decision, belief, or goal stated in the present tense.

Agency. The ability to initiate an action; the intrinsic capacity to act in the world, to do things in a way that is neither predetermined nor random.

Ambivalence. Contradictory attitudes or feelings toward an action or uncertainty about which approach to follow. Ambivalence can occur when personal values are not aligned with desired change or are evidenced by any uneasiness or unwillingness of a commitment to change.

Appreciate. To fully understand a situation and to recognize the full worth of a person and their life experiences and valuing what is shared.

Appreciative Inquiry (AI). A relational process based on affirmation, appreciation, and dialogue.

Authentic advocacy. Actions taken on behalf of others that arise from a deep alignment of one's beliefs, values, and behaviors. This connotes an "egoless" engagement for the purpose of benefitting and serving/sourcing from soul's purpose/soul's wisdom (Rushton, 2018).

Authenticity. Consistency with a person's beliefs, values, and actions, which demonstrate what one believes to be their truth.

Bearing witness. Being present with another. A state and skills that are achieved and learned through reflective practice (relaxation, prayer, meditation, nature walks) that can shift an experience of separateness to one of connection; bearing witness involves developing the qualities of stillness in order to be present for others.

Caring. The moral ideal of nursing consisting of human-to-human attempts to protect, enhance, and preserve human dignity, integrity, and wholeness by assisting a person to find meaning in illness, suffering, pain, and existence (Watson, 2007).

Change talk. Expressions by an individual, which indicate intent to change or how they will follow through with desired goals; this change talk can be subtle and culturally specific.

Code of Ethics (Nursing). A list of nine provisions that makes explicit the primary goals, values, and obligations of the nursing profession and expresses its values, duties, and commitments to the society of which it is a part. In the United States, nurses abide by and adhere to the American Nurses Association (ANA) *Code of Ethics for Nurses With Interpretive Statements* (ANA, 2015b). At the global level, nurses follow the International Council of Nurses Code of Ethics (ICN, 2012).

Compassion. The ability to be present for all levels of suffering with no need to "fix" the suffering; it is the tenderness of the heart in response to suffering.

Compassion fatigue. A state that arises when nurses experience weariness and fatigue because of their long exposure to suffering and situations that are physically or emotionally traumatizing, without adequate support, or ability to calm and care for themselves.

Competency. An expected and measurable level of nursing performance that integrates the art and science of nursing knowledge, skills, and judgment, based on established scientific knowledge and expectations for nursing practice.

Core values. Belief of convictions that direct behavior and support one's purpose in life.

Cultural knowledge and congruent care. The concepts, language, and acknowledgement of healthcare consumers, families, and communities that connect to their ethnic and/or social health-related values, beliefs, and traditional practices.

Decisional balance. Weighing the pros and cons that are associated with a change behavior.

Deep listening. The communication between two or more individuals in which the conventional division of self and ego are transcended by a sense of indivisible unity between everyone involved. Deep listening involves being present, allowing space, and being focused with intention to understand what another person is expressing or not expressing.

Discrepancy. Lack of engagement or inconsistency with a decision or action steps toward a healthier behavior or goal.

Ecosystem. A system or a group of interconnected elements formed by the interaction of individuals, groups, communities, and organisms with their environment.

Embodied awareness. Nurse Coaches strive to become aware of bodily sensations or messages. They are consciously in the present moment as change is taking place in the present.

Emotional intelligence (EI). The ability to perceive emotion in self and others; the ability to use emotions as a source of information; the ability to comprehend the complex relationships among emotions; and the ability to manage emotions to achieve desired outcomes. EI is concerned with understanding self and others and being able to relate to others. EI requires attunement to social norms and is a learned capability.

Empathy. Understanding the feelings of another; the capacity to vicariously experience the feelings or thoughts of another without having to have those thoughts or feelings expressed explicitly.

Empirical knowing. The science of nursing that focuses on formal expression, replication, and validation of scientific competence in nursing education and practice. It is expressed in models and theories and can be integrated into evidence-based practice. Empirical indicators are accessed through the known senses that are subject to direct observation, measurement, and verification.

Energy. Life force; a sense of being stimulated to act.

Engagement. Actions individuals must take to obtain great benefit from the healthcare services available to them (Center for Advancing Health, 2010, p. 2).

Environment. The context of habitat within which all living systems participate and interact, including climate, the physical body, and its physical habitat along with the cultural, psychological, social, and historical influences. This includes both the external physical space and the person's internal physical, mental, emotional, social, and spiritual experience, seen and unseen vibrations, frequencies, and energy pattern.

Environmental determinants of health. Any external agent (biological, chemical, physical, social, or cultural) that can be linked to a change in health status of individuals and communities that is involuntary. For example, breathing unwanted secondhand smoke is an environment determinant of health, whereas active tobacco smoking is a behavioral determinant. These determinants are the natural environment, such as plants, weather, or climate change; built environment, such as buildings or transportation; worksites, schools, and recreational settings; housing, homes, and neighborhoods; exposure to toxic substances and other physical hazards; physical barriers, especially for people with disabilities; and aesthetic elements, such as good lighting, trees, or benches (Health People.gov, 2018).

Equanimity. The spacious stillness that accepts things as they are; the invitation to see the present moment as the truth of our human condition and to be present to our experience.

Ethical knowing. The moral knowledge in nursing that focuses on behaviors, expressions, and dimensions of both morality and ethics. Ethical knowing includes valuing and clarifying situations to create formal moral and ethical behaviors intersecting with legally prescribed duties. Ethical knowing emphasizes respect for the person, the family, and the community that encourages connectedness and relationships that enhance attentiveness, responsiveness, communication, and moral action.

Ethics. The basic underlying concept of the unity and integral wholeness of all people and all of nature that is identified and pursued by finding unity and wholeness within one's self and within humanity. In this framework, acts are not performed for the sake of law, precedent, or social norms, but rather from a desire to do good freely in order to witness, identify, and contribute to unity.

Evidence-based practice. The process by which healthcare practitioners make clinical decisions using the best philosophy and theories, research evidence, clinical expertise, and patient preferences within the context of available resources.

Evidence-informed practice. Concept developed to include and go beyond the standard set by quantitative evidence-based practice in order to incorporate a more comprehensive set of clinical data that supports a thorough holistic assessment from subjective, anecdotal, or common sense sources.

Generative moments. Experiences in which an individual is inspired toward change, growth, and a vision.

Global health. Worldwide focus on the health of all people with a priority of achieving equality, reducing disparities, and protecting against global threats that are not confined to national borders—local to global; it is a global commons, a bridge across boundaries, and a path to world peace (Nightingale Initiative for Global Health, n.d.).

Graduate level-prepared nurse coach. Nurses who have completed master's education in administration, education, or other related fields and pursue beyond basic level nurse coaching.

Healing. A lifelong journey seeking harmony and balance in one's own life and in family, community, and global relations. Healing involves those physical, mental, social, and spiritual processes of recovery, repair, renewal, and transformation that increase wholeness and often (though not invariably) order and coherence.

Healing process. A continual journey of changing and evolving one's self through a life that is characterized by the awareness and resolution of patterns that support or are challenges/barriers to health and healing. This journey may be done alone or in a healing community. The healing process may occur until a person's final breath.

Healing relationships. The quality and characteristics of interactions between two or more people toward harmony and balance such as interactions that involve empathy, caring, love, warmth, trust, confidence, credibility, competence, honesty, courtesy, respect, sharing expectations, and open communication for a heart-to-heart connection.

Health. A defined state or process in which the nurse, person, family, group, community or population experiences a sense of growth, well-being, harmony, and unity such that subjective experiences about health, health beliefs, and values are honored; a process of becoming an expanding consciousness; may occur in the presence or absence of disease or injury.

Health and Wellness Nurse Coach-Board Certified (HWNC-BC). An AHNCC Board-Certified Holistic Nurse (HN-BC or AHN-BC) who has also passed the AHNCC Nurse Coach Certification Examination.

Health intervention. An act performed for, with, or on behalf of a person or population to assess, improve, maintain, promote, or modify health functioning or health conditions.

Health promotion. Activities and preventive measures to facilitate growth, promote health, increase well-being, that actualize human potential of people, families, communities, society, and populations. Examples include; immunizations, fitness/exercise programs, breast self-exam, appropriate nutrition, relaxation, stress management, social support, prayer, meditation, healing rituals, cultural practices, and promotion of environmental health and safety.

Healthcare consumer. The individual person, family, group, community, or population who is the focus of attention, and to whom the nurse coach is providing services as sanctioned by state regulatory bodies.

Holistic. Based on an understanding that each person is an interconnected unity and that physical, mental, emotional, social, and spiritual factors need to be included in any health interventions. The whole is a system that is greater than the sum of its parts.

Holistic communication. A free flow of verbal and nonverbal interchange between and among people and significant beings such as pets, nature, and God/Life Force/Absolute/Transcendent that explores meaning and ideas leading to mutual understanding and growth.

Human caring. The moral ideal of nursing in which the nurse brings one's entire self into a relationship with the whole self of the healthcare consumer in order to protect the person's vulnerability, preserve their humanity and dignity, and reinforce the meaning and experience of oneness and unit.

Human energy field (HEF). A luminous field of energy that comprises a person, extends beyond the physical body, and is in a continuous mutual process with the environment. HEF is a vital energy that is recognized by its unique pattern; HEF is dynamic, creative, nonlinear, unpredictable, and flows in lower and higher vibration.

Human health experience. An individual's personal experiences and expressions (both internal and external awareness) that include one's worldview related to health, health beliefs, attitudes, values, cultural beliefs, sexual orientation, and life's continuum from birth to death and beliefs in the afterlife.

Illness. A subjective experience of symptoms that a person may describe with specific meaning (physical, mental, emotional, spiritual, environmental cultural, and or energetic) that result in imbalance and disharmony; illness may not be synonymous with disease.

Integral. A comprehensive synthesizing framework or multidimensional perspective. An integral approach addresses all levels of human experience (subjective and objective; individual and collective) in a combined, synergistic manner.

Integrative. An approach that puts the client at the center and addresses the whole person and full range of physical, emotional, mental, social, spiritual, and environmental influences that affect health; includes the client's personalized action plan to maintain optimal health behaviors and human flourishing, and to heal illness and disease.

Intention. The conscious act of stating an action, approach, or future state of being which can augment or facilitate health and well-being.

International Classification of Health Interventions (ICHI). A classification system of healthcare procedure codes that has been under development since 2007 by the World Health Organization (WHO), and contains approximately 7,000 intervention codes for use by interdisciplinary providers.

Interpersonal collaboration. Engagement with other healthcare professionals, community leaders, thought leaders, and healthcare consumers as appropriate to improve the health of people, nations, and countries. Also see *Transdisciplinary dialogue.*

Intuition. The perceived internal knowing of things and events without the conscious use of rational processes; using all the senses to receive and process information.

Lifestyle. A manner of living that reflects a person's values and attitudes.

Meaning. That which is signified, indicated, referred to, or understood; more specifically *philosophical meaning* refers to—meaning that depends on the symbolic connections that are grasped by reason; *psychological meaning refers to*—meaning that depends on connections that are experienced through intuition or insight; *spiritual meaning refers to*—the meaning around the ultimate issues, questions, and concerns of "Who am I?" "What is my soul's purpose?" How am I part of the interconnected web of life?" (Dossey, 2003).

Mindfulness. Inner capacity of cultivating a nonjudgmental awareness and understanding of our experience as it is arising in order to create present moment awareness; this space allows for moments of solitude so that our inner hidden parts and patterns may emerge and time to sit with what emerges (suffering, fear, joy, happiness, etc.).

Moral injury. An emotional state that occurs when a nurse is faced with an ethical dilemma that occurs when a nurse is unable to provide the care that he or she believes is right or best for the healthcare consumer (i.e., policies and procedures, lack of resources or communication, conflicting perspectives or worldviews, patient choice/belief, etc.). This situation can cause the nurse to experience feelings of anxiety, powerlessness, or depression.

Moral intelligence. The mental capacity to apply universal human principles, (integrity, responsibility, compassion, forgiveness, etc.) to personal values, goals, and actions.

Moral resilience. A process aimed at restoring, preserving, or deepening moral integrity and ultimately cultivating the sustained capacity for principled moral action; embedded in this process is the capacity to engage in a process of moral repair (Rushton, 2018, pg. 126).

Moral suffering. An anguish experienced as a threat to our composure, our integrity, the fulfillment of our intentions, and more deeply as a frustration to the concrete meaning that we have found in our personal experience (Reich, 1989).

Motivation. The process that drives a person to make choices and take action.

Motivational Interviewing (MI). An intervention strategy for changing behavior. The central purpose of MI is to help healthcare consumers explore and eventually resolve ambivalence in reference to a current health behavior; emphasizes a person's choice and responsibility and can be used in a variety of clinical settings.

Motivator. A reason for action; can be external or internal.

Not knowing: The capacity to use healing presence, to be spontaneously open to the moment with no preconceived answers or anticipated outcomes.

It engages authenticity, mindfulness, openness, receptivity, surprise, mystery, and discovery with self and others in the subjective space and the intersubjective space that allows for new solutions, possibilities, and insights to emerge. It acknowledges the patterns that may not be understood that may manifest related to various situations or relationships.

Nurse Coach. A baccalaureate-prepared registered nurse who integrates coaching competencies into any setting or specialty area of practice to facilitate a process of change or development that assists individuals or groups to realize their potential. See also *Nurse Coach-Board Certified (NC-BC) and Health and Wellness Nurse Coach-Board Certified (HWNC-BC)*.

Nurse Coach Board Certified (NC-BC). A baccalaureate-prepared registered nurse who has successfully passed the American Holistic Nurses Association Credentialing Corporation (AHNCC) Nurse Coach Certification Examination.

Nurse Coach Leadership. An individual contributor who embodies strengths, purpose, values, ethics, and vision and future expectations that can be shared with others in interprofessional collaboration; this includes opening to intuitive insights and inner wisdom, which allows caring, compassion, purpose, authenticity, humility, and integrity to manifest (Dossey & Luck, 2015).

Nurse Coaching. A skilled, purposeful, result-oriented, and structured relationship and person-centered interaction with a healthcare consumer that is provided by a baccalaureate-prepared registered nurse for the purpose of promoting achievement of a person's goals.

Nurse Coaching process. A critical thinking model and process that involves *six* steps that may occur simultaneously: (1) Establishing relationship and identifying readiness for change (Assessment); (2) Identifying opportunities, issues, and concerns (Diagnosis); (3) Establishing person-centered goals (Outcomes); (4) Creating the structure of the coaching interaction (Planning); (5) Empowering and motivating the individual to reach goals (Intervention); and (6) Assisting individual to determine the extent to which goals were achieved (Evaluation).

Nursing Interventions Classification (NIC). A standardized comprehensive classification or taxonomy of interventions that nurses perform including both independent and collaborative as well as direct and indirect care.

Nursing Outcomes Classification (NOC). A standardized comprehensive taxonomy of frequently identified outcomes and measurable responses to nursing interventions.

Nursing process. A critical thinking model that involves *six* steps that may occur simultaneously: (1) Assessment; (2) Diagnosis; (3) Outcomes; (4) Planning; (5) Implementation; and (6) Evaluation.

Omaha System (OS). A research-based, standardized healthcare terminology, recognized by the American Nurses Association, used by multidisciplinary practitioners, and designed to describe client care; includes an assessment component (Problem Classification Scheme), a care plan/service component (Intervention Scheme), and an evaluation component (Problem Rating Scale for Outcomes). Users represent the continuum of care, and more than 22,000 multidisciplinary clinicians use Omaha System point-of-care software in the United States and other countries (www. Omaha system.org).

Open-ended questions (OEQ). Questions in which there is no simple yes or no response; OEQ questions encourage reflection and meaningful responses.

Outcome-based practice. Based on the individual's value, perception, and meaning of the outcome, the nurse coach and individual determine how the outcome(s) will be measured.

Outcome expectations. Development of situation specific mutually agreed upon scales with a series of activities listed in order of difficulty, which are behavior specific and used as the foundation for assessing self-care abilities. Interventions that are relevant for the individual can then be developed based on outcome expectations.

Patterns of knowing. A mode of inquiry that encompasses empirical, ethical, personal, aesthetic and socio-political assessment and evaluation, appropriate to the generation to provide diverse sources of data for evidence-based nursing practice.

Person. An individual, healthcare consumer, client, patient, family member, significant other, support person, or community member who engages with the nurse coach.

Person-centered care. The human caring process in which the nurse coach gives full attention and intention to honor the whole person, family, groups, or community. Person-centered care involves respecting individual values and choices and ensuring continuity of care. It is a time of exploring the experience and concerns of the healthcare consumer and others while reinforcing wholeness and unity.

Personal knowing. The nurse's dynamic process and awareness of wholeness that focuses on the synthesis of perceptions and being with self. Personal knowing may be developed through art, meditation, dance, music, stories, and other forms of creative expression. Insights gained through dreams and other reflective practices that reveal symbols, images, and other connections also influence one's interior environment.

Praxis. The use of theory in practice that explores the interrelationships of theory, practice, and research, and informs healthcare policy.

Presence. The condition of being consciously and compassionately in the present moment with another, believing in the person's inherent wholeness, whatever the current situation; the essence of nursing care; the gift of self. Presence involves approaching an individual or a situation in a way that shows respect, honor and wholeness and enters into a shared field of consciousness that promotes growth and healing.

Presence as a nursing intervention. Combines attributes, such as, intentionality, mutuality, centeredness, and attention. Presence transforms experiences, adds a deeper, more powerful dimension, reduces anxiety, and promotes a nurturing atmosphere. Presence is a way of being that involves connection so that growth and healing are promoted for self and others.

Problem-solving. Discovering, analyzing, and solving problems using a systematic approach based on perceived deficit.

Quality of life. A broad concept and subjective measure of the overall well-being of an individual, person, family, group, community, or population that incorporates all aspects of life.

Reflection. Inner awareness of our thoughts, feelings, judgments, beliefs, and perceptions.

Reflective practice. A process of learning to be in the present moment that guides inner knowing and development of wholeness and unity; reflective practice informs the nurse coach on ways to be with another. It is Attentive, Critical, Exploratory, Iterative (ACEI); underlying Conceptual Frame (CF); View of Change (VC); and Self (S) (Sadlon, 2018).

Reflective practitioner. A healthcare professional who engages in reflective practice to more deeply examine one's story (interiority and exteriority) about life's journey (meaning, struggles, strengths, purpose, mission, beliefs, values, ethics, etc.) as well as how to collaborate with others toward healthy people living on a healthy planet.

Relationship-centered care. A process model of caregiving that is based in a vision of community in which relationships (the patient–practitioner, community–practitioner, and practitioner–practitioner) are considered essential, and each person shares a unique set of responsibilities where all involved feel honored and valued.

Resilience. The process of adapting well in the face of adversity, trauma, tragedy, threats, or significant sources of stress such as family and relationship problems, serious health problems, or workplace and financial stressors.

Resistance. Reactive "push back" with comments, behavior, or attitude that interferes with a desire to change health behaviors. Sources of resistance can include such factors as fear, doubt, feelings of overwhelm or lack of knowledge.

Scope of Nursing Practice. The description of the *who, what, where, when, why,* and *how* of nursing practice that addresses the range of nursing practice activities common to all registered nurses. When considered in conjunction with the ANA *Nursing: Scope and Standards of Professional Nursing Practice* and the ANA *Code of Ethics with Interpretive Statements, for Nurses,* this comprehensively describes the competent level of nursing common to all registered nurses.

Self-assessment. A centered, dynamic, and ongoing informal caring process where one uses inherent wisdom to identify personal patterns, concerns, and opportunities; formal assessments may occur through the use of standardized wellness tools in collaboration with a nurse coach or healthcare professional who provides additional data to the individual, who then engages in self-assessment.

Self-care. Tending to (or attention to) the mind, body, spirit through activities such as creative expression, physical exercise, time in nature, mindfulness, and healthy eating; occurs throughout the lifespan as one uses compassion-focused awareness, reflective choices, and self-determined actions and behaviors in a meaningful way.

Self-confidence. A person's belief in one's capacity to make a behavioral change.

Self-development. A process of taking personal responsibility for one's learning and development, often involving self-reflection, self-assessment, self-evaluation, and self-care as an integral process.

Self-efficacy. The personal belief that one has the capability of initiating change with a sense of empowerment and ability to make healthful choices that leads to enduring change.

Self-esteem. The belief that one has personal value and self-worth.

Self-evaluation. The exploration of a person's understanding, experiences, and behaviors; may include the measurement of self-care actions with the use of a tool or a specific goal to determine, if, how and why, desired, or specific outcomes have been achieved.

Self reflection. An inner awareness of a person's thoughts, feelings, judgments, beliefs, and perception that opens the process for the intentional and conscious use of self as a therapeutic instrument in the healing process (McElligott, 2015).

Skill acquisition (skill attainment). The ability to integrate the knowledge, skills (technical and nontechnical) and attitudes necessary to provide safe patient care. The nurse coach progresses through five stages of proficiency: novice, advanced beginner, competent, proficient, and expert (Benner, 1984).

Social determinants of health. The economic and social conditions under which individuals live that affect their health; disease and illness are often a result of detrimental social, economic, and political forces. Examples of social determinants are availability of resources to meet daily needs (safe housing educational and job opportunities, living wages, etc.); healthy foods, social norms and attitudes, (discrimination, racism, etc.); exposure to crime, violence, and social disorder (the presence of trash; social support and interactions); access to mass media and emerging technologies, (the internet, cell phones); socio-economic conditions, concentrated poverty, quality schools; transportation options; public safety; and residential segregation (Health People.gov, 2018).

Sociopolitical knowing. Integrating important contextual variables of social, economic, geographic, cultural, political, historical, and other key factors in theoretical, evidence-based practice and research. This pattern includes informed critique and social justice for the voices of the underserved in all areas of society along with protocols to reduce health disparities.

Soul pain. The experience of an individual who has become disconnected and alienated from the deepest and most fundamental aspects of one's self.

Soul's purpose. Arises from a felt sense of profound meaning, intention, and focus about one's life and work.

Spiritual intelligence. The recognition that physical reality is embedded within a larger, multidimensional reality with which we interact, knowingly or unknowingly. This larger reality includes and transcends the ego and the physical body. Spiritual intelligence involves the ability to act with compassion and wisdom, while maintaining inner and outer peace, regardless of circumstances. Spiritual intelligence includes the ability to access one's deepest meanings and highest motivations.

Standards. Authoritative statements defined and promoted by the nursing profession by which quality of practice, education, and service can be evaluated.

Standards of Practice. Standards that describe a competent level of nursing care as demonstrated by the nursing process. *See also* Nursing process.

Standards of Professional Nursing Practice. Authoritative statements of the duties that all registered nurses, regardless of role, population, or specialty are expected to perform competently (ANA, 2015a).

Standards of Professional Performance. Standards that describe a competent level of behavior in the professional role.

Story. A dynamic process where the storyteller (individual, family, group) embraces the telling of a happening or connected series of happenings; narrative meaning usually combines human actions or events that affect the storyteller, thus impacting the whole person.

Strengths. Preexisting patterns of thought, feeling, and behavior that are authentic, energizing, and lead to best potentials and possibilities.

Suffering. An individual's experience of struggle based on a reinforced story around anxiety, distress, or pain. Suffering can manifest as behavioral, emotional, mental, moral, physical, social, and/or spiritual signs of distress; can be anguish experienced—internal and external—as a threat to one's composure, integrity, sense of self, or the fulfillment of expectations.

Transdisciplinary dialogue. An approach where interprofessional colleagues explore deep meaning that engages the human spirit and spiritual concerns, connections, ideas, visioning, and evolving possibilities rather than competition between and among.

Transpersonal. A personal understanding that is based on one's experiences of temporarily transcending or moving beyond one's usual identification with the limited biological, historical, cultural, and personal self at the deepest and most profound levels of experience possible. From this perspective, the ordinary, biological, historical, cultural, and personal self is seen as an important but only a partial manifestation or expression of this much greater something that is one's deeper origin and destination. Transpersonal is that which transcends the limits and boundaries of individual ego identities and possibilities to include acknowledgment and appreciation of something greater.

Unknowing. A state of being that is open to not knowing.

Values clarification. An intervention in which an individual can discover, clarify and define one's own values by assessing, exploring, and evaluating the effect of their own personal values on decision making.

Vicarious trauma. The painful emotional impact that nurses, first responders, and others experience as a result of hearing about or bearing witness to the vulnerability, pain, fear, and suffering of trauma survivors and their loved ones.

Vulnerability. The reality of the human condition that recognizes that all are subject to change and loss at any time. The awareness that our physical life is transitory.

Wellbeing. A general term for the condition of an individual or group, and their social, economic, psychological, spiritual, environmental, and medical state; based on the idea that the way each person thinks and feels about their life is meaningful and important.

Wellness. A desirable quality of life that provides satisfaction; a multidimensional state of existence experienced as well-being; integrated, congruent functioning aimed toward reaching one's highest potential.

Wisdom. Sourcing action from the deepest place within so that motivation for action and challenges may emerge.

Worldview. The way an individual sees oneself in the universe, living with self and others; worldview reflects beliefs, values, relationships, moral and ethical reasoning, and connectedness with all living things.

*Note. Definitions adapted from *Holistic Nursing: A Handbook for Practice* (2016); ANA's *Nursing: Scope and Standards of Practice* (2015) and *Nurse Coaching: Integrative Approach for Health and Wellbeing* (2015). Used with permission.

References and Bibliography

Accenture.com. (2019). Retrieved from https://www.accenture.com.ng.en

Ahmad, M., Al-Rimawi, R., Masadeh, A., & Atoum, M. (2015). Workplace violence by patients and their families against nurses: Literature review. *International Journal of Nursing and Health Science, 2*(4), 46–55.

Amaya, M., Melynk, B. M., & Neale, S. (2018). Environmental wellness. *American Nurse Today, 13*(9), 94–95.

American Association of Colleges of Nursing (AACN). (2011). *Fact sheet.* Retrieved from http://www.aacn.nche.edu/Media/FactSheets/nursfact.htm.

American Association of Colleges of Nursing (AACN). (2008). *The essentials of baccalaureate education for professional nursing practice.* Retrieved from http://www.aacn.nche.edu/Education/pdf/BaccEssentials08.pdf.

American Holistic Nurses Credentialing Corporation (AHNCC). (2017). *Nurse coach core essentials.* Retrieved from https://www.ahncc.org/wp-content/uploads/2018/12/FINAL-REVISED-NC-Core-Essentials-DOC-4-12-2017.pdf.

American Holistic Nurses Credentialing Corporation (AHNCC). (n.d.). *Nurse coach certification examination handbook and credentialing and application.* Retrieved from https://ptcny.com/pdf/AHNCC-Nurse-Coach.pdf.

American Holistic Nurses Association & American Nurses Association (AHNA/ANA). (2013). *Holistic nursing: Scope and standards of practice* (2nd ed.). Silver Spring, MD: Author.

American Hospital Association. (2018). Nurse watch: Nurses again top Gallup Poll of trusted professions and other nurse news. Retrieved from https://www.aha.org/news/insights-and- analysis/2018-01-10-nurse-watch-nurses-again-top-gallup-po

American Nurses Association. (n.d.). *Healthy Nurse Healthy Nation Grand Challenge.* Retrieved from http://www.healthynursehealthynation.org.

American Nurses Association (ANA). (2015a). *Nursing: Scope and standards of nursing practice,* (3rd ed.). Silver Spring, MD: Author.

American Nurses Association (ANA). (2015b). *Code of ethics for nurses with interpretive statements.* Washington, DC: Author.

American Nurses Association & American Holistic Nurses Association (ANA/AHNA). (2019). *Holistic nursing: Scope and standards of practice* (3rd ed.). Silver Spring, MD: Nursesbooks.org.

American Nurses Credentialing Center. (2017). *2019 Magnet© Recognition Program.* Silver Spring, MD: Author.

American Nurses Credentialing Corporation. (n.d.). Retrieved from https://nursingworld.org/ancc/.

American Organization of Nursing Executives. (n.d.). Retrieved from https://www.aha.org/websites/2012-10-11-aone.

Antonovsky, A. (1996). The salutogenic model as a theory to guide health promotion. *Health Promotion International, 11*(1), 11–18.

Aoki, T., Yamamoto, Y., Ikenoue, T., Urushibara-Miyachi, Y., Kise, M., Fujinuma, Y., & Fukuhara, S. (2018). Social isolation and patient experience in older adults. *Annals of Family Medicine, 16*(5), 393–398.

Armstrong, C., Wolever, R. Q., Manning, L., Elam, R., Moore, M., Frates, P., Duskey, H., Anderson, C., Curtis, R. L., Masemer, S., & Lawson, K. (2013). Group health coaching: Strengths, challenges, and next steps. *Global Advances in Health and Medicine, 2*(3), 95–102.

Assagioli, R. (1991). *Transpersonal development: The dimension beyond psychosynthesis.* London: HarperCollins.

Assagioli, R. (1974). *Act of will.* New York: Viking.

Assagioli, R. (1965). *Psychosynthesis.* New York: Penguin.

Atkinson, P. A., Martin, C. R., & Rankin, J. (2009). Resilience revisited. *Journal of Psychiatric and Mental Health Nursing, 16,* 137–145.

Bandura, A. (1977). Self-efficacy: Toward a unifying theory of behavioral change. *Psychological Review, 84*(2), 191, 215.

Bark, L. (2011). *The wisdom of the whole: Coaching for joy, health, and success.* San Francisco, CA: Create Space.

Bark, L. (2001). *Developing and maintaining a healthy culture using coaching principles.* San Francisco, CA: Author.

Barrett, E. A. M. (2003). Update on a measure of power as knowing participation in change. In O. L. Strickland & C. DiIorio (Eds.), Vol. 4. *Measurement of nursing outcomes: Focus on patient/client outcomes* (pp. 21–39). New York: Springer.

Barrett, E. A. M. (1983). *An empirical investigation of Martha E. Rogers' principle of helicy: The relationship of human field motion and power.* Unpublished doctoral dissertation, New York University, New York.

Baumann, L. A., Baker, J., & Elshaug, A. G. (2018). The impact of electronic health record systems of clinical documentation times: A systematic review. *Health Policy Amsterdam, Netherlands, 122*(8), 827–836.

Beck, D. M., Dossey, B. M., & Rushton, C. H. (2019). Florence Nightingale's legacy for the 21st Century: Global activism, advocacy, and transformation. In Kreitzer, M. J., & Koithan, M. *Integral Nursing* (2nd ed., pp. 678–688). New York: Oxford University Press.

Becker, M. H. (1974). The health belief model and sick role behavior. *Health education monographs, 2*(4), 409–419.

Bell, J. A. (2013). Five generations in the nursing workforce: Implications for nursing professional development. *Journal for Nurses in Professional Development, 29*(4), 205–210.

Benner P. (1985). The oncology clinical specialist: An expert coach. *Oncology Nursing Forum, 12*(2), 40–44.

Benner P. (1984). *Novice to expert: Excellence and power in clinical nursing practice.* Menlo Park, CA: Addison-Wesley.

Benzo, R. P., Kramer, K. M., Hoult, J. P., Anderson, P. M., Begue, I. M., & Seifert, S. J. (2018). Development and feasibility of a home pulmonary rehabilitation program with health coaching. *Respiratory Care, 63*(2), 131–140.

Bindman, A. B. (2013). Using the national provider identifier for health care workforce evaluation. *Medicare & Medicaid Research Review, 3*(3), E1–E10.

Black, J. T., Romano, P. S., Banafsheh, S., Auerbach, A., Ganiats, T. G., Greenfield, S., Kaplan, S. H., Ong, M. K., & The BEAT-HF Research Group. (2014). A remote monitoring and telephone nurse coaching intervention to reduce readmissions among patients with heart failure: Study protocol for the Better Effectiveness After Transition-Heart Failure (BEAT-HF) randomized controlled trial. *Trials*. Retrieved from http://www.trialsjournal.com/content/15/1/124.

Blackwell, D. L., & Clarke, T. C. (2018). State variation in meeting the 2008 federal guidelines for both aerobic and muscle-strengthening activities through leisure-time physical activity among adults aged 18–64: United States, 2010–2015. *National Health Statistics Reports, 112*(6), 1–22. Retrieved from https://www.cdc.gov/nchs/data/nhsr/nhsr112.pdf.

Bodenheimer, T., & Sinsky, C. (2014). From triple aim to quadruple aim: Care of the patient requires care of the provider. *The Annals of Family Medicine, 12*(6), 573–576. doi: 10.1370/afm.1713.

Booth, J. (2015). Motivational interviewing: Helping patients make lifestyle changes. *Nurse.Com, 25*(12), 22–27. Retrieved from https://www.nurse.com/ce/motivational-interviewing.

Brookings Institute. (2016). Retrieved from https://www.brookings.edu/series/building-healthy-neighborhoods/.

Brown, T. (2018). *Enhanced interstate nurse licensure compact implemented.* Retrieved from https://www.medscape.com/viewarticle/891782.

Butler, S., & Diaz, C. (2017). Nurses as intermediaries in the promotion of community health: Exploring their roles and challenges. *Building Healthy Neighborhoods Series: Brookings Institute.*

Cable, S., & Graham, E. (2018). Leading better care: An evaluation of an accelerated coaching intervention for clinical nursing leadership development. *Journal of Nurse Management, 6*(5), 605–612.

Cacioppo, J. T., & Cacioppo, S. (2018). The growing problem of loneliness. *The Lancet, 391*(10119), 426. doi.org/10.1016/S0140-6736(18)30142-9.

Cangelosi, J. (2020). Comparison of Millennials, Generation X, and Baby Boomers Attitudes Toward Preventive Health Information: A Social Media Emphasis.

Carpenter, C. J. (2010). A meta-analysis of the effectiveness of health belief model variables in predicting behavior. *Health Communication, 25*(8), 661–669.

Carper, B. A. (1978). Fundamental patterns of knowing in nursing. *Advances in Nursing Science, 1*(1), 13–23.

Cassel, C. K. (2018). Can retail clinics transform health care? *Journal of American Medical Association, 319*(18), 1855–1856.

Center for Advancing Health. (2010). A new definition of patient engagement: What is engagement and why is it important (p. 2). Washington D.C.

Centers for Disease Control and Prevention. (2018). Suicide rates rising across the U.S.: Comprehensive prevention goes beyond a focus on mental health concerns. Retrieved from https://www.cdc.gov/media/releases/2018/p0607-suicide-prevention.html.

Centers for Disease Control and Prevention. (2016). Chronic diseases: The leading causes of death and disability in the United States. Retrieved from https://www.cdc.gov/chronicdisease/overview/index.htm.

CGFNS International. Retrieved from http://www.cgfns.org/sections/about/.

Chenoweth, L., Gallagher, R., Sheriff, J. N., Donoghue, J., & Stein-Parbury, J. (2008). Factors supporting self-management in Parkinson's disease: Implications for nursing practice. *International Journal of Older People Nursing, 3*(3), 187–193.

Clavelle, J. T., & Prado-Inzerillo, M. (2018). Inspire others through transformational leadership. *American Nurse Today, 13*(11), 39–41.

Clayton, M. F., Dean, M., & Mishel, M. (2018). Theories of uncertainty in illness. In Smith, M. J., & Liehr, P. R. (Eds.). *Middle range theory for nursing* (4th ed., pp. 49–82). New York: Springer Publishing Company.

Collier, R. (2017). Electronic health records contributing to physician burnout. *CMAJ: Canadian Medical Association Journal, 189*(45), E1405–E1406. https://doi.org/10.1503/cmaj.109-5522.

Cooperrider, D., Whitney, D. D., Stavros, J. M., & Stavros, J. (2008). *The appreciative inquiry handbook: For leaders of change.* Berrett-Koehler Publishers.

Cormack, C. L., Jensen, E., Durham, C. O., Smith, G., & Dumas, B. (2018). The 360-degree evaluation model: A method for assessing competency in graduate nursing students. A pilot research study. *Nurse Education Today, 64,* 132–137.

Cowling, W. R. (2001). Unitary appreciative inquiry. *Advances Nursing Science, 23*(4), 32–48.

Cowling, W. R. (2000). Healing as appreciating wholeness. *Advances in Nursing Science, 22*(3), 16–32.

Cumming, R. (2018). Nurse leader talks about respectful, healthy work environments. *American Nurse Today, 13*(4), 23.

CVS Health. (2018). CVS to acquire Aetna. Retrieved from CVS health.com https://cvshealth.com/newsroom/press-releases/cvs-health-acquire-aetna-combination-provide-consumers-better-experience.

Davidson, A. W., Ray, M. A., & Turkel, M. C. (Eds.). (2011). Nursing, caring, and complexity science: For human environment well-being. Springer Publishing Company.

Davidson, O. B., Feldman, D. B., & Margalit, M. (2012). A focused intervention for 1st-year college students: Promoting hope, sense of coherence, and self-efficacy. *Journal of Psychology Interdisciplinary and Applied, 146*(3), 333–352.

Davis, L. A. (2015a). Motivational interviewing and nonviolent communication. In B. M. Dossey, S. Luck, & B. G. Schaub. *Nurse coaching: Integrative approaches for health and wellbeing* (pp. 313–325). North Miami, FL: International Nurse Coach Association.

Davis, L. A. (2015b). Appreciative inquiry. In B. M. Dossey, S. Luck, & B. G. Schaub. *Nurse coaching: Integrative approaches for health and wellbeing* (pp. 327–334). North Miami, FL: International Nurse Coach Association.

Davis, L. A. (2015c). Nurse coaching education. In B. M. Dossey, S. Luck, & B. G. Schaub. *Nurse coaching: Integrative approaches for and wellbeing* (pp. 351–366). North Miami, FL: International Nurse Coach Association.

Deci, E. L., & Ryan, R. M. (2002). Overview of self-determination theory: An organismic dialectical perspective. *Handbook of self-determination research,* 3–33.

Delaney, C., & Bark, L. (2019). The experience of holistic nurse coaching for patients with chronic conditions. *Journal of Holistic Nursing.* https://ournals/sagepub.com/doi/full.

Delaney, C., Barrere, C., & Bark, L. (2020). A metaphor analysis of patients' with chronic conditions experiences with holistic nurse coaching. *Holistic Nursing Practice, 34*(1), 24–34.

DiClemente, C. C., & Prochaska, J. O. (1998). *Toward a comprehensive, transtheoretical model of change: Stages of change and addictive behaviors.* New York: Plenum Press.

Donner, G. J., & Wheeler, M. M. (2009). *Coaching in nursing: An introduction.* Indianapolis, IN: International Council of Nurses & Sigma Theta Tau International.

Dossey, B. M. (2020). Theory of integral nursing. In M. C. Smith (Ed.). *Nursing theories and nursing practice* (5th ed. pp. 211–234). Philadelphia: F. A. Davis.

Dossey, B. M. (2016). Nursing: Holistic, integral, and integrative—local to global. In C. C. Barrere, M. A. Blaszko Helming, D. Shields, & K. Avino (Eds.). B. M. Dossey, & L. Keegan (Original Authors). *Holistic nursing: A handbook for practice* (7th ed., pp. 3–52). Burlington, MA: Jones and Bartlett Learning.

Dossey, B. M. (2015a). Theory of integrative nurse coaching. In B. M. Dossey, S. Luck, & B. G. Schaub. *Nurse coaching: Integrative approaches for health and wellbeing* (pp. 29–49). North Miami, FL: International Nurse Coach Association.

Dossey, B. M. (2015c). Stories, strengths, and the nurse coach 5-Step process. In B. M. Dossey, S. Luck, & B. G. Schaub. *Nurse coaching: Integrative approaches for health and wellbeing* (pp. 85–108). North Miami, FL: International Nurse Coach Association.

Dossey, B. M. (2010). *Florence Nightingale: Mystic, visionary, healer.* Commemorative Edition. Philadelphia: F. A. Davis.

Dossey, B. M. (2008). Theory of integral nursing. *Advances in Nursing Science, 33*(1), E52–73.

Dossey, B. M., Luck, S., & Schaub, B. G. (2015). *Nurse coaching: Integrative approaches for health and wellbeing* (pp. 387–404). North Miami, FL: International Nurse Coach Association.

Dossey, L. (2003). Samueli conference of definitions and standards of healing research: Working definitions and terms. *Alternative Therapies in Health and Medicine, 9*(3); A11.

Dossey, B. M., Rosa, W., & Beck, D. M. (2019). Nursing and the sustainable development goals (SDGs): From Nightingale to now. *American Journal of Nursing, 119*(5), 40–45.

Dube, A., Freeman, E., & Reich, M. (2010). *Employee replacement costs.* Retrieved from http://irle.berkeley.edu/files/2010/Employee-Replacement-Costs.

Dunlap, J. J. (2019). How Can We Practice Mindful Presence? *Journal of Christian Nursing, 36*(3), 196.

Dyess, S. M., Prestia, A. S., Marquit, D. E., & Newman, D. (2018). Self-care for nurse leaders in acute care environment reduces perceived stress: A mix-methods pilot study merits further investigation. *Journal of Holistic Nursing, 36*(1), 79–90.

Dyess, S. M., Sherman, R., Opalinski, A., & Eggenberger, T. (2017). Structured coaching programs to develop staff. *The Journal of Continuing Education in Nursing, 48*(8), 373–378.

Engebretson, J. (2016). Cultural diversity and care. In C. C. Barrere, M. A. Blaszko Helming, D. Shields, & K. Avino (Eds.). B. M. Dossey, & L. Keegan (Original Authors). *Holistic nursing: A handbook for practice* (7th ed., pp. 439–464). Burlington, MA: Jones and Bartlett Learning.

Englander, R., Cameron, T., Ballard, A. J., Dodge, J., Bull, J., & Aschenbrener, C. A. (2013). Toward a common taxonomy of competency domains for the health professions and competencies for physicians. *Academic Medicine, 88*(8), 1088–1094.

Erickson, E., Tomlin, E., & Swain, M. A. (2019). *Modeling and role-modeling: A theory and paradigm for nursing.* In M. C. Smith, & D. Gullett. *Nursing theories and nursing practice* (5th ed., pp. 183–209). Philadelphia: F. A. Davis.

Erickson, H. L., Erickson, M. E., Southard, M. E., Brekke, M. E., Sandor, M. K., & Natschke., M. (2016). A proactive innovation for health care transformation: Health and wellness nurse coaching. *Journal of Holistic Nursing, 34*(1), 44–55.

Erickson, E., Tomlin, E., & Swain, M. A. (2009). *Modeling and role-modeling: A theory and paradigm for nursing.* Englewood Cliffs, NJ: Prentice-Hall.

Eriksson, I., Lindblad, M., Moller, U., & Gillsijo, C. (2018). Holistic health care: Patients' experiences of health care provided by an advanced practice nurse. *International Journal of Nursing Practice, 24*(1), e12603. Retrieved from https://www.ncbi.nlm.nih.gov/pmc/articles/PMC5813192.

Fahlberg, B., & Roush, T. (2019). Mindful presence: Being "with" in our nursing care. *Nursing 2019, 46*(3), 14–15.

Fathi, J. T., Modin, H. E., & Scott, J. D. (2017). Nurses advancing telehealth services in the era of healthcare reform. *Online Journal of Issues in Nursing, 22*(2).

Fawcett, J. (1995). *Analysis and evaluation of conceptual models of nursing* (3rd ed.). Philadelphia: F. A. Davis.

Fawcett, J., & DeSanto-Madeya, S. (2005). Peplau's theory of interpersonal relations. Contemporary nursing knowledge (2nd ed., pp. 528–552). Philadelphia, PA: FA Davis.

Fazio, S., Edwards, J., Miyamoto, S., Henderson, S., Dharmar, M., & Young, H. M. (2019). More than A1C: Types of success among adults with type-2 diabetes participating in a technology-enabled nurse coaching intervention. *Patient Education and Counseling, 102*(1), 106–112.

Flinter, M., Hsu, C., Cromp, D. A., Ladden, M. J. D., & Wagner, E. H. (2017). Registered nurses in primary care: Emerging roles and contributions to team-based care in high-performing practices. *Journal of Ambulatory Care Management, 40*(4), 287–96.

Foreman, K. J., Marquez, N., Dolgert, A., Fukutaki, K., Fullman, N., McGaughey, M., & Brown, J. C. (2018). Forecasting life expectancy, years of life lost, and all-cause and cause-specific mortality for causes of death: Reference and alternative scenarios for 2016–40 for 195 countries and territories. *The Lancet, 392*(10159), 2052–2090. Retrieved from https://www.cdc.gov/media/releases/2018/p0607-suicide-prevention.html.

Fowler, M. D. M. (2015). *Guide to the code of ethics for nurses with interpretative statements: Development, interpretation, and application,* 2nd ed. Silver Spring, MD: Nursebooks.org.

Frey, L. M., & Ratliff, J. L. (2018). The personal and professional experiences of integrative Nurse Coach certificate program graduates: A pilot study. *Journal of Holistic Nursing, 36*(2), 134–144.

Frisch, N. C., & Potter, P. (2016). Nursing theory in holistic nursing practice. In C. C. Barrere, M. A. Blaszko Helming, D. Shields, & K. Avino (Eds.). B. M. Dossey, & L. Keegan (Original Authors). *Holistic nursing: A handbook for practice* (7th ed., pp. 111–120). Burlington, MA: Jones and Bartlett Learning.

Fronstin, P. (2018). Consumer Engagement in Health Care Among Millennials, Baby Boomers, and Generation X: Findings from the 2017 Consumer Engagement in Health Care Survey. *EBRI Issue Brief,* (444).

Fry, R. (2018). Millennials projected to overtake Baby Boomers as America's largest generation. Pew *Research Center,* 1.

Gagné, M., & Deci, E. L. (2005). Self-determination theory and work motivation. *Journal of Organizational behavior, 26*(4), 331–362.

Gallup. (2020). Nurses again outpace other professions for honesty, ethics. Retrieved from https://news.gallup.com/poll/274673/nurses-continue-rate-highest-honesty-ethics.aspx.

Gebser, J. (1985). *The Ever Present Origin,* trans. Noel Barstad with Algis Mickunas. Ohio University press, Athens, OH.

Gelinas, L. (2018). Listening as a caring competency. *American Nurse Today, 13*(10), 4.

Ghani, A. A. (2019). The Impact of the nurse licensing compact on inter-state job mobility in the United States. *OECD Economic Survey of the United States: Key Research Findings,* 105.

Gillespie, B. M., Chaboyer, W., & Wallis, M. (2007). Development of a theoretically derived model of resilience through concept analysis. *Contemporary Nurse, 25*(1–2), 124–135.

Goble, K. L., Knight, S. M., Burke, S. C., Carawan, L. W., & Wolever, R. Q. (2017). Transformative change to 'a new me': A qualitative study of clients' lived experience with integrative health coaching. *Coaching: An International Journal of Theory, Research and Practice, 10*(1), 18–36.

Godfrey, M. M., Anderson-Gare, B., Nelson, E. C., Nilsson, M., & Ahlstrom, G. (2014). Coaching interprofessional health care improvement teams: The coachee, the coach and the leader perspectives. *Journal of Nursing Management, 22*(4), 452–464.

Gordon, P. A. (2017). Exploring generational cohort work satisfaction in hospital nurses. *Leadership in Health Services, 30*(3), 233–248.

Grof, S. (1992). *Theoretical and empirical foundations of transpersonal psychology.* Revised paper presented at the Twelfth International Transpersonal Conference entitled Science, Spirituality, and the Global Crisis: Toward A World with A Future, June 20–25, 1992, Prague, Czechoslovakia.

Gusovsky, D. (2016). *CNBC Americans consume vast majority of the world's opioids.* Retrieved from https://www.cnbc.com/2016/04/27/americans-consume-almost-all-of-the-global-opioid-supply.html.

Gustin, L. W. (2018). Being mindful as a phenomenological attitude. *Journal of Holistic Nursing, 36*(3), 272–279.

Haddad, L. M., & Toney-Butler, T. J. (2018). Nursing shortage. StatPearls. Retrieved from https://www.ncbi.nlm.nih.gov/books/NBK493175/.

Hampton, D. C., & Keys, Y. (2016). Generation Z students: Will they change our nursing classrooms? *Journal of Nursing Education and Practice, 7*(4), 111.

Hartweg, D. L. (2014). Dorothea Orem's self-care deficit nursing theory. In M. E. Parker, & M. C. Smith, *Nursing theories and nursing practice* (4th ed., pp. 121–145). Philadelphia: F. A. Davis.

Haudenschield, J., & Blachek, J. (2018). *Next generation healthcare.* Brentwood, TN: AIL Press.

Havaei, F., MacPhee, M., & Susan Dahinten, V. (2016). RNs and LPNs: Emotional exhaustion and intention to leave. *Journal of Nursing Management, 24*(3), 393–399.

Hawkins, P. (2012). *Creating a coaching culture: Developing a coaching strategy for your organization.* London: McGraw-Hill Education UK.

Hayes, E., & Kalmakis, K. A. (2007). From the sidelines: Coaching as a nurse practitioner strategy for improving health outcomes. *Journal of the American Academy of Nurse Practitioners, 19*(11), 555–562.

Healthy Nurse Healthy Nation. (n.d.). Retrieved from https://www.nursingworld.org/practice-policy/work-environment/health-safety/healthy-nurse-healthy-nation/.

Healthy People Framework 2030. (n.d.). Retrieved from https://www.healthypeople.gov/2020/About-Healthy-People/Development-Healthy-People-2030/Framework.

Hess, D. R., Dossey, B. M., Southard, M. E., Luck, S., Schaub, B. G., & Bark, L. (2013). *The art and science of nurse coaching: A provider's guide to coaching scope and competencies.* Silver Spring, MD: Nursesbooks.org.

Hoelzel, B. K., Carmody, J., Vangel, M., Congleton, C., Yerramsetti, S. M., & Gard. (2011). Mindfulness practice leads to increases in regional brain gray matter density. *Psychiatry Research: Neuroimaging, 191*(1), 36–43.

Hope, S., & Rosa, W. (2018). Holistic care of the spirit: The use of entheogens in patients with advanced serious illness. *Beginnings, 38*(4), 18–21.

Horton-Deutsch, S., & Anderson, J. (2018). *Caritas coaching: A journey toward transpersonal caring for informed moral action in healthcare.* Indianapolis, IN: Sigma Theta Tau International.

Hrabe, D., Melynk, B. M., & Neale, S. (2018). Spiritual wellness: A journey towards wellness. *American Nurse Today, 13*(10), 24–26.

Huang, Y. J., Parry, M., Zeng, Y., Luo, Y., Yang, J., & He, G. P. (2017). Examination of a nurse-led community-based education and coaching intervention for coronary heart disease high-risk individuals in China. *Asian Nursing Research (Korean Society Nursing Science), 11*(3), 187–193.

Institute for Healthcare Improvement (IHI). (2018). *The IHI triple aim.* Retrieved from http://www.ihi.org/engage/initiatives/tripleaim/Pages/default.aspx.

Institute of Medicine. (2012). *Living well with chronic illness: A call to action.* Washington, DC: The National Academies Press.

Institute of Medicine, Committee on the Robert Wood Johnson Foundation Initiative on the Future of Nursing. (2011). *The future of nursing: Leading change, advancing health.* Washington DC: National Academies Press.

International Coach Federation. (2019). ICF core competencies. Retrieved from https://coachfederation.org/core-competencies.

International Council of Nurses. (n.d.). Retrieved from http://www.icn.ch/.

International Nurse Coach Association (INCA). (n.d.). Retrieved from http://www.inursecoach.com.

Interprofessional Education Collaborative Expert Panel. (2011). *Core competencies for interprofessional collaborative practice: Report of an expert panel.* Washington, D.C.: Interprofessional Education Collaborative.

Jarrad, R., Hammad, S., Shawashi, T., & Mahmoud, N. (2018). Compassion fatigue and substance use among nurses. *Annals of General Psychiatry, 17*(1), 13.

Johns, C. (Ed.). (2017). *Becoming a reflective practitioner.* John Wiley & Sons.

Johns, C. (1995). Framing learning through reflection within Carper's fundamental ways of knowing in nursing. *Journal of Advanced Nursing, 22*(2), 226–234.

Jordan, M. (2013). Health coaching for the underserved. *How to be a Health Coach: An Integrative Wellness Approach.* San Rafael, CA: Global Medicine Enterprises, Inc.

Jowsey, T., Dennis, S., Yen, L., Mofizul Islam, M., Parkinson, A., & Dawda, P. (2016). Time to manage: Patient strategies for coping with an absence of care coordination and continuity. *Sociology of Health & Illness, 38*(6), 854–873.

Kabat-Zinn, J. (1991). *Full catastrophe living: Using the wisdom of your body and mind to face stress, pain, and illness.* New York: Delta Trade Paperbacks.

Kantor, J. (2017). High turnover costs way more than you think. Retrieved from https://www.huffingtonpost.com/julie-kantor/high-turnover-costs-way-more-than-you-think_b_9197238.html.

Kauffman, C. (2006). Positive psychology: The science at the heart of coaching. In D. R. Stober & A. M. Grant (Eds.), *Evidence based coaching handbook: Putting best practices to work for your clients* (pp. 219–253). Hoboken, NJ: John Wiley & Sons Inc.

Kearns, K., Dee, A., Fitzgerald, A. P., Doherty, E., & Perry, I. J. (2014). Chronic disease burden associated with overweight and obesity in Ireland: The effects of a small BMI reduction at population level. *BMC Public Health, 14*(1), 143. Retrieved from https://www.ncbi.nlm.nih.gov/pmc/articles/PMC3929131/. doi: 10.1186/1471-2458-14-143.

Kegan, R., & Lahey, L. L. (2009). *Immunity to change: How to overcome it and unlock the potential in yourself and your organization.* Boston: Harvard Business School Publishing.

Langeland, E., Wahl, A. K., Kristoffersen, K., & Hanestad, B. R. (2007). Promoting coping: Salutogenesis among people with mental health problems. *Issues in Mental Health Nursing, 28,* 275–295.

Lee-Kwan, S. H., Moore, L. V., Blanck, H. M., Harris, D. M., & Galuska, D. (2017). Disparities in state-specific adult fruit and vegetable consumption—United States, 2015. *MMWR. Morbidity and Mortality Weekly Report, 66*(45), 1241. Retrieved from https://www.cdc.gov/media/releases/2017/p1116-fruit-vegetable-consumption.html.

Leininger, M. (2006). Cultural care diversity and universality theory and evolution of the ethnonursing method. In M. M. Leininger & M. R. McFarland (Eds.). *Culture care diversity and universality: A worldwide nursing theory* (2nd ed., pp. 1–42). Sudbury, MA: Jones & Bartlett Learning.

Leihr, P. R., & Smith, M. J. (2018). Story theory. In M. J. Smith, & P.R. Leihr. (Eds.). *Middle range theor for nursing* (4th ed., pp. 241–264). New York: Springer Publishing Company.

Leininger, M. (2002). *Transcultural nursing: Theories, concepts and practices* (3rd ed.). New York: McGraw Hill.

Lillienfeld, E., Nicholas, P. K., Breakey, S., & Corless, I. (2018). Addressing climate change through a nursing lens within the framework of the United Nations Sustainable Development Goals. *Nursing Outlook, 66*(5), 482–494.

Luck, S. (2015a). Nutritional health. In B. M. Dossey, S. Luck, & B. G. Schaub. *Nurse coaching: Integrative approaches for health and wellbeing* (pp. 147–163). North Miami, FL: International Nurse Coach Association.

Luck, S. (2015b). Environmental health. In B. M. Dossey, S. Luck, & B. G. Schaub. *Nurse coaching: Integrative approaches for health and wellbeing* (pp. 165–176). North Miami, FL: International Nurse Coach Association.

Luck, S., & Dossey, B. M. Cultural perspectives and rituals of healing (2015). In B. M. Dossey, S. Luck, & B. G. Schaub. *Nurse coaching: Integrative approaches for health and wellbeing* (pp. 335–347). North Miami, FL: International Nurse Coach Association.

Luszczynska, A., Scholz, U., & Schwarzer, R. (2005). The general self-efficacy scale: Multicultural validation studies. *The Journal of Psychology: Interdisciplinary and Applied, 139*(5), 439–457.

Makary, M., & Daniel, M. (2016). Medical error-the third leading cause of death in the US. *British Medical Journal, 353*(i2139). doi: 10.1136.

Malerba, B. P., Richman, D. A., Koziak, A., & Radler, R. (2018). *The status of telemedicine reimbursement: States' efforts to incentivize providers to utilize telehealth technologies.* Retrieved from https://www.americanbar.org/groups/health law/publications/ aba_health_esource/2016-2017/december2017/telehealth/.

Mallock, K., & Porter-O'Grady, T. (2005). *The quantum leader: Applications for the new world of work.* Sudbury, MA: Jones and Bartlett.

Marrone, S. R. (2017). The art of knowing: Designing a nursing professional development program based on American nurses' experiences of providing care to Arab Muslims. *Journal of Nursing Education and Practice, 7*(7), 104–111.

Martin, K. S. (2009). The Omaha System: A key to practice, documentation, and information management. WB Saunders Co.

Martinez, A. J. S. (2016). Managing workplace violence with evidence-based interventions: A literature review. *Journal of Psychosocial Nursing and Mental Health Services, 54*(9), 31–36.

Masterson, L. (2018). CMS unveils strategy to improve rural healthcare. *Health Care Dive.* Retrieved from https://www.healthcaredive.com/news/ cms-unveils-strategy-to-improve-rural-healthcare/523092/.

Mauriello, L. M., Johnson, S. S., & Prochaska, J. M. (2017). Meeting patients where they are at: Using a stage approach to facilitate engagement. In *Practical strategies and tools to promote treatment engagement* (pp. 25–44). New York: Springer Publishing Company.

McCarthy, R., D., Feuerlicht, E., Ohn, B., & Silverstone, Y. (2018). Accenture-developing a culture of coaching leadership. Retrieved from https://www.accenture.com/us-en/ insight-outlook-developing-culture-of-coaching-leadership.

McCraty, R., & Childres, D. (2010). Coherence: Bridging personal, social, and global health. *Alternative Therapies in Health and Medicine, 16*(4), 10–24.

McDermott-Levy, R., Leffers, J., & Mayaka, J. (2018). Ethical principles and guidelines of global health nursing practice. *Nursing Outlook, 66*(5), 473–481.

McElligott, D., Eckardt, S., Dossey, B. M., Luck, S., & Eckardt, P. (2018). Instrument development of integrative health and wellness assessments. *Journal of Holistic Nursing, 36*(4), 374–384.

McElligott, D. (2015). Nurse coach self-development. In B. M. Dossey, S. Luck, & B. G. Schaub. *Nurse coaching: Integrative approaches for health and wellbeing* (pp. 407–417). North Miami, FL: International Nurse Coach Association.

McNally, K., & Cunningham, L. (2010). *The Nurse Executive's Coaching Manual.* Indianapolis, IN: Sigma Theta Tau International.

Mechcatie, E. (2019). The top nursing news stories of 2018. *American Journal of Nursing, 119*(1), 19.

Melynk, B. M., & Neale, S. (2018a). Physical wellness: A must for sustained energy. *American Nurse Today, 13*(2), 28–29.

Melynk, B. M., & Neale, S. (2018b). Emotional wellness. *American Nurse Today, 13*(3), 61–63.

Melynk, B. M., & Neale, S. (2018c). Intellectual wellbeing. *American Nurse Today, 13*(5), 24–25.

Melynk, B. M., & Neale, S. (2018d). Social wellness: Nurture your relationships. *American Nurse Today, 13*(7), 42–44.

Meretoja, R., Isoaho, H., & Leino-Kilpi, H. (2004). Nurse competence scale: Development and psychometric testing. *Journal of Advanced Nursing, 47*(2), 124–133.

Merriam-Webster Dictionary. (2019). Definition of coach. Retrieved from https://www.merriam-webster.com/dictionary/coach

Miller, W. R., & Rollnick, S. (2002). *Motivational interviewing: Preparing people for change* (2nd ed.). New York, NY: Guilford Press.

Miller, W. R., & Rollnick, S. (2012). *Motivational interviewing: Helping people change.* New York, NY: Guilford Press.

Mishel, M. H. (1990). Reconceptualization of the uncertainty in illness theory. *Image: The Journal of Nursing Scholarship, 22*(4), 256–262.

Mishel, M. H. (1988). Uncertainty in illness. *Image: The Journal of Nursing Scholarship, 20*(4), 225–232.

Munhall, P. L. (1993). Unknowing: Toward another pattern of knowing in nursing. *Nursing Outlook, 41*(3), 125–128.

Murphy, S., Jiaquan Xu, B., Kochanek, K. M. A., & Arias, E. *Mortality in the United States Centers for Disease Control and Prevention* (2018). Retrieved from https://www.cdc.gov/nchs/products/databriefs/db328.htm.

Nagle, M. A. (2018). Global perspective on creating space to nurture wholeness in nursing. *Beginnings, 38*(2), 10–11, 24–25.

National Committee on Quality Care. (n.d.). Retrieved from https://www.ncqa.org.

National Consortium for the Credentialing of Health and Wellness Coaches Progress Report---July, 2011. (2011). Retrieved from http://www.wellcoaches.com/images/pdf/progressreport-nationalteam-jul-2011.pdf.

National Consortium of Telehealth Resource Centers. (n.d.). Retrieved from https://www.telehealthresourcecenter.org.

National Council of State Boards of Nursing. (n.d.). Retrieved from https://www.ncsbn.org/index.htm.

Natschke, M. (2015). A proactive innovation for health care transformation: Health and wellness nurse coaching. *Journal of Holistic Nursing, 34*(1), 44–55.

Neuman, B., & Fawcett, J. (Eds.). (2010). *The Neuman systems model* (5th ed). Upper Saddle River, NJ: Pearson.

Newberg, A., & Waldman, M. (2017). *How enlightenment changes your brain.* New York: Penguin.

Newman, M. A. (1999). *Health as expanding consciousness* (2nd ed.). St. Louis, MO: C.V. Mosby.

Newman, M. A. (1994). *Health as expanding consciousness*. St. Louis, MO: C.V. Mosby.

Newman, N., Fletcher, R., Kalogeropoulos, A., Levy, D. A., & Nielsen, R. K. (2017). Reuters Institute Digital News Report. Retrieved from https://reutersinstitute.politics.ox.ac.uk/sites/default/files/Digital%20News%20Report%202017%20web_0.pdf.

Newell, S., & Jordan, Z. (2015). The patient experience of patient-centered communication with nurses in the hospital setting: A qualitative systematic review protocol. *JBI Database System Rev Implement Rep.*, *13*(1), 76–87. Retrieved fromhttps://www.ncbi.nlm.nih.gov/pubmed/26447009.

Niesen, C. R., Kraft, S. J., & Meiers, S. J. (2018). Use of motivational interviewing by nurse leaders: Coaching for performance, professional development, and career goal setting. *The Health Care Manager, 37*(2), 183–192.

Nightingale, F. (1893). Sick-nursing and health-nursing. In B. Coutts (Ed.), *Woman's Mission* (pp. 184–205). London, England: Sampson, Low, Marston.

Nightingale, F. (1860). *Notes on nursing: What it is and what it is not.* London, England: Harrison.

Nightingale, F. (1859). *Notes on hospitals.* London, England: John W. Parker.

Nightingale Declaration for a Healthy World. (n.d.). Retrieved from https://www.nighvision.net/nightingale-declaration.html.

Nightingale Initiative for Global Health. (n.d.). Retrieved from HYPERLINK "http://www.nighvision.net/" \t "_blank" http://www.nighvision.net

Norcross, J. C. (2012). Changeology: 5 steps to realizing your goals and resolutions (Vol. 35, No. 6). Simon and Schuster.

Nothwehr, F. (2007). Self-efficacy and its association with use of diet-related behavioral strategies and reported dietary intake. *Health Education and Behavior, 35*(5), 698–706.

Nurse Compact License. (n.d.). Retrieved from https://www.ncsbn.org/nurse-licensure-compact.htm.

Nursing NOW. (n.d.). Retrieved from https://www.nursingnow.org.

Occupational Safety and Health Administration. (n.d.). Workplace violence in healthcare: Understanding the challenge. OSHA 3826, 12/2105. Retrieved from https://www.osha.gov/Publications/OSHA3826.pdf.

Orem, D. E. (1971). *Nursing concepts of practice.* New York, NY: McGraw Hill.

Ornish, D. (1990). *Dr. Dean Ornish's Program for Reversing Heart Disease.* New York: Ballentine Books.

Palabindala, V., Pamarthy, A., & Jonnalagadda, N. R. (2016). Adoption of electronic health records and barriers. *Journal of Community Hospital Internal Medicine Perspectives, 6*(5). https://doi.org/10.3402/jchimp.v6.32643.

Patient Protection and Affordable Care Act, H. R. 3590. Pub. 1. No. 111-148. (2010). Retrieved from https://www.congress.gov/bill/111th-congress/house-bill/3590.

Parse, R. R. (1995). *Illuminations: The human becoming theory in practice and research.* New York, NY: National League for Nursing Press.

Parse, R. R. (1981). *Man-living-health: A theory of nursing.* New York: John Wiley & Sons.

Pekurinen, V., Willman, L., Virtanen, M., Kivimäki, M., Vahtera, J., & Välimäki, M. (2017). Patient aggression and the wellbeing of nurses: A cross-sectional survey study in psychiatric and non-psychiatric settings. *International Journal of Environmental Research and Public Health, 18*(10). pii: E1245. doi: 10.3390/ijerph14101245.

Peplau, H. E. (1952). *Interpersonal relations in nursing.* New York, NY: GP Putnam's Sons.

Perry, D. J. (2004). Self-transcendence: Lonergan's key to integration of nursing theory, research, and practice. *Nursing Philosophy, 5*(1), 67–74.

Petri, G., Atanasova, S., & Kamin, T. (2017). Effective clinical practice. *Patient Empowerment and Healthcare, 4*(6), 256–62.

Potter, P., & Frisch, N. C. (2013). The nursing process. In Dossey, B. M., & Keegan, L. *Holistic nursing: A handbook for practice* (6th ed., pp. 145–160). Burlington, MA: Jones & Bartlett Learning.

Priani, S. M., Hong, O. S., & Chen, J. (2018). Lifestyle and health-related outcomes of U. S. hospitals nurses: A systematic review. *Nursing Outlook, 66*(1), 66–76.

Prochaska, J. O., Norcross, J. C., & DiClemente, C. C. (1994). *Changing for good: A revolutionary six-stage program for overcoming bad habits and moving your life positively forward.* New York, NY: Harper Collins.

Professional Testing Corporation. (n.d.) Retrieved from https://ptcny.com.

Quinn, J. (2016). Transpersonal human caring and healing. In C. C. Barrere, M. A. Blaszko Helming, D. Shields, & K. M. Avino (Eds). B. M. Dossey, & L. Keegan (Original Authors). *Holistic nursing: A handbook for practice* (7th ed., pp. 101–109). Burlington, MA: Jones and Bartlett Learning.

Ray, M. A. (2016). *Transcultural caring dynamics in nursing and health care.* FA Davis.

Reich, W. T. (1989). Speaking of suffering: A moral account of compassion. *Soundings, 72*(1), 83–108.

Resnick, B. (2018). The theory of self-efficacy. In Smith, M. J., & Liehr, P. R. (Eds.). *Middle range theory for nursing* (4th ed., pp. 215–240). New York: Springer Publishing Company.

Rigg, K. K., Monnat, S. M., & Chavez, M. N. (2018). Opioid-related mortality in rural America: Geographic heterogeneity and intervention strategies. *International Journal of Drug Policy, 57,* 119–129.

Robert Wood Johnson Foundation. (2013). *Transforming care at the bedside toolkit.* Retrieved from http://www.rwf.org/qualityequalityproduct.jsp.

Roberts, S. (2010). Listening to (and saving) the world's languages. *New York Times.* Retrieved from https://www.nytimes.com/2010/04/29/nyregion/29lost.html.

Rogers, M. E. (1994). The science of unitary human beings: Current perspectives. *Nursing Science Quarterly, 7*(1), 33–35.

Rogers, M. E. (1970). *An introduction to the theoretical basis of nursing.* Philadelphia, PA: F. A. Davis.

Rollnick, S., Miller, W. R., & Butler, C. C. (2008). *Motivational interviewing in healthcare: Helping patient change behavior.* New York, NY: Guilford Press.

Rosa, W., Horton-Deutsch, S., & Watson, J. (2019). *A handbook for caring science.* New York: Springer Publishing Company.

Rosa, W. E., Upvall, M. J., Beck, D. M., & Dossey, B. M. (2019). Nursing and sustainable development: Furthering the global agenda in uncertain times. *Online Journal of Issues in Nursing, 24*(2), DOI: 10.3912/OJIN.

Rosa, W. (2018). Transcultural holism: A global literacy for health and healing. *Beginnings, 38*(2), 12–15.

Rosa, W. (2017). One mind – one health – one planet: A pledge to planetary citizenship. In Rosa, W. (Ed.). *A new era in global health: Nursing and the 2030 sustainable development agenda* (pp. 517–520). New York, NY: Springer Publishing Company.

Rosa, W. E., Hope, S., & Matso, M. (2018). Palliative nursing and sacred medicine: A holistic stance on ethoeogens, healing, and spiritual care. *Journal of Holistic Nursing, 37*(1), 100–106.

Ross, A., Brooks, A. T., Yang, L., Touchton-Leonard, K., Raju, S., & Bevans, M. (2018). Results of a national survey of certified nurse coaches with implications for advanced practice nurses. *Journal of the American Association of Nurse Practitioners, 30*(5), 251–261.

Rosselli, M., & Vanni, D. (2014). Roberto Assagioli and Carl Gustav Jung. *Journal of Transpersonal Psychology, 46*(1), 7–34.

Roy, C. (2009). *The Roy adaptation model* (3rd ed.). Upper Saddle River, NJ: Prentice-Hall Health.

Rushton, C. H. (2018). *Moral resilience: Transforming moral suffering in healthcare.* New York: Oxford University Press.

Ryan, R. M., & Deci, E. L. (2017). *Self-determination theory: Basic psychological needs in motivation, development, and wellness.* Guilford Publications.

Ryan, R. M., & Deci, E. L. (2000). Self-determination theory and the facilitation of intrinsic motivation, social development, and well-being. *American Psychologist, 55*(1), 68.

Sadlon, P. (2018). The process of reflection: A principle-based concept analysis. *Nursing Forum, 53*(3), 364–368.

Sandle, T. (2017). Boomers, Genxers, Millenials, GenZ Healthcare Expectations. http://www. digitaljournal.com/life/health/boomers-gen-xers-millennials-gen-z-healthcare-expectations/ article/497028#ixzz5bWIMjPZw.

Sang, M. J., & Benevente, V. (2016). Health coaching in nurse practitioner-led group visits for chronic care. *The Journal of Nurse Practitioners, 12*(4), 258–264.

Schablon, A., Wendeler, D., Kozak, A., Nienhaus, A., & Steinke, S. (2018). Prevalence and consequences of aggression and violence towards nursing and care staff in Germany: A survey. *International Journal of Environmental Research and Public Health, 15*(15), 1274.

Schaub, B. G. (2016). Vulnerable and spiritual: Utilizing the process of Transpersonal Nurse Coaching. In W. Rosa (ed.). *Nurses as leaders: Evolutionary visions of leadership* (pp. 377–392). New York: Springer Publishing.

Schaub, B. G. (2015). Awareness and choice. In B. M. Dossey, S. Luck and B. G. Schaub. *Nurse coaching integrative approaches for health and wellbeing* (pp. 211–237). North Miami FL: International Nurse Coach Association.

Schaub, B. G., & White, M. B. (2015). Transpersonal coaching. *Beginnings, 35*(4), 14–16.

Schaub, R., & Schaub, B. G. (2013). *Transpersonal development. Cultivating the human resources of peace, wisdom, purpose and oneness.* Huntington, NY: Florence Press.

Schaub, B. G., Luck, S., & Dossey, B. M. (2012). Integrative nurse coaching for health and wellness. *Alternative and Complementary Therapies, 18*(1), 14–20.

Schaub, R., & Schaub, B. G. (2009). *The end of fear: A spiritual path for realists.* Carlsbad, CA: Hay House.

Schaub, B., & Schaub, R. (1997). *Healing addictions: The vulnerability model of recovery.* Albany, NY: Delmar Publishers.

Schaub, R., & Simon, B. (2018). Easing diabetes distress. Integrative Practitioner, Nov. 9. https://www.integrativepractitioner.com/topics/mind-body/easing-diabetes-distress

Seligman, M. E. P. (2006). *Learned optimism: How to change your mind and your life.* New York: Free Press.

Seligman, M. E., & Csikszentmihalyi, M. (2014). Positive psychology: An introduction. In *Flow and the foundations of positive psychology* (pp. 279–298). Springer.

Sherman, R. O. (2018). Building your resilience. *American Nurse Today, 13*(9), 26–28.

Sherwood, G., & Barnsteiner, J. (Eds.). (2017). *Quality and safety in nursing: A competency approach to improving outcomes.* John Wiley & Sons.

Shields, D., & Stout Shaffer, S. (2016). Self-development. The foundation of holistic care. In In C. C. Barrere, M. A. Blaszko Helming, D. Shields, & K. Avino (Eds). B. M. Dossey, & L. Keegan (Original Authors). *Holistic nursing: A handbook for practice* (7th ed., pp. 683–702). Burlington, MA: Jones and Bartlett Learning.

Sigma Theta Tau International. Retrieved from http://www.nursingsociety.org/aboutus/mission/ Pages/factsheet.aspx.

Smith, M. C. (2019). Theory of unitary caring. In M. C. Smith, & D. Gullett. *Nursing theories and nursing practice* (5th ed., pp. 493–502). Philadelphia: F. A. Davis.

Smith, M. J., & Leihr, P. R. (2014). Story theory. In M. J. Smith, & P. R. Leihr (Eds.). *Middle range theory for nursing* (3rd ed.) New York: Springer Publishing Company.

Snyderman, R., & Dinan, M. (2010). Improving health by taking it personally. *JAMA: Journal of the American Medical Association, 303*(4), 363–364.

Southard, M. E. (2018). *Communication in Health Care.* Western Schools. Brockton, MA.

Southard, M. E. (2016). Maintenance of nursing certification: Ensuring holistic nursing competency. *Beginnings, 36*(4), 26–27.

Southard, M. E. (2003). *Standards of practice for nurse coaching training: An integrative approach to wellness coaching.* Copyright. Author.

Southard, M. E., Bark, L., Erickson, M., & Monsen, K. A. (2017). Feasibility of using the Omaha System to represent nurse coaching practice. *Kontakt, 19*(1), E4–E11.

Southard, M. E., Bark, L., & Hess, D. R. (2016). Facilitating change: Motivational interviewing and appreciative inquiry. In C. C. Barrere, M. A. Blaszko Helming, D. Shields, & K. Avino (Eds). B. M. Dossey, & L. Keegan (Original Authors). Holistic Nursing: A handbook for practice (7th ed., pp. 551–556). Burlington, MA: Jones and Bartlett Learning.

Spence, G. B., & Oades, L. G. (2011). Coaching with self-determination theory in mind: Using theory to advance evidence-based coaching practice. *International Journal of Evidence-Based Coaching and Mentoring, 9*(2), 37–55.

Stevanin, S., Palese, A., Bressan, V., Vehviläinen-Julkunen, K., & Kvist, T. (2018). Workplace-related generational characteristics of nurses: A mixed-method systematic review. *Journal of Advanced Nursing, 74*(6), 1245–1263.

Stewart-Lord, A., Baillie, L., & Woods, S. (2017). Health care staff perceptions of a coaching and mentoring programme: A qualitative case study evaluation. *International Journal of Evidence Based Coaching and Mentoring, 15*(2), 70–85.

Sutin, A. R., Stephan, Y., Luchetti, M., & Terracciano, A. (2018). Loneliness and risk of dementia. *Journal of Gerontology: Series B*, gby112. Retrieved from https://doi.org/10.1093/geronb/gby112.

Taylor, H., & McElligott, D. (2015). Nurse coaching and research. In B. M. Dossey, S. Luck, & B. G. Schaub (Eds.), *Nurse coaching: Integrative approaches for health and wellbeing* (pp. 367–385). North Miami, FL: International Nurse Coach Association.

United Nations Sustainable Development Goals 2030 Agenda. (2019). Retrieved from https://sustainabledevelopment.un.org/sdgs.

Upton, K. V. (2018). An investigation into compassion fatigue and self-compassion in acute medical care hospital nurses: A mixed methods study. *Journal of Compassionate Health Care, 5*(1), 7.

U.S. Department of Health and Human Services, Office of Disease Prevention and Health Promotion. (n.d.). *Introducing healthy people 2020.* Retrieved from http://www.healthypeople.gov/2020/about/default.aspx.

U.S. Nursing Workforce in 2018 and Beyond. (2018). *Journal of Nursing Regulation, 8*(4), S3–S6.

van Houwelingen, C. T., Moerman, A. H., Ettema, R. G., Kort, H. S., & ten Cate, O. (2016). Competencies required for nursing telehealth activities: A Delphi-study. *Nurse Education Today, 39*, 50–62.

Watson Caring Science Institute. (n.d.). *Caritas coaching education program.* Watson, J. (1985). *Nursing: Human science and human caring—A theory of nursing.* Norwalk, CT: Appleton & Lange.

Watson, J. (2007). *Nursing human science and human care: A theory of nursing.* Sudbury, MA: Jones and Bartlett.

Watson, R., Stimpson, A., Topping, A., & Porock, D. (2002). Clinical competence assessment in nursing: A systematic review of the literature. *Journal of Advanced Nursing, 39*(5), 421–431.

Wellard, S., J., Lillibridge, J., Beanland, C. J., & Lewis, M. (2003). Consumer participation in acute care settings: An Australian experience. *International Journal of Nursing, 9*(4), 255–260.

White, J. (1995). Patterns of knowing: Review, critique, and update. *Advances in Nursing Science, 17*(2), 73–86.

Whitmore, J. (2002). *Coaching for Performance: The Principles and Practice of Coaching and Leadership FULLY REVISED 25TH ANNIVERSARY EDITION.* Hachette UK.

Whitney, D., & Cooperrider, D. (2011). *Appreciative inquiry: A positive revolution in change.* ReadHowYouWant.Com.

Wilson, M. (2009). Complexity theory. *Whitireia Nursing Journal, 16*, 18–24.

Wolever, R. Q., Simmons, L. A., Sforzo, G. A., Dill, D., Kaye, M., Bechard, E. M., Southard, M. E., & Yang, N. (2013). A systematic review of the literature on health and wellness coaching: defining a key behavioral intervention in healthcare. *Global Advances in Health and Medicine, 2*(4), 38–57.

WHO Collaborating Centers (WHOCCs) for Nursing and Midwifery Development. (n.d.). Retrieved from http://www.globalnetworkwhocc.com.

Wong, K. (2018). Fighting the effects of nurse fatigue. *American Nurse Today, 12*(5), 40–41.

World Health Organization. (2009). Patient empowerment and health care. Retrieved from https://www. ncbi. nlm. nih. gov/books/NBK144022.

Wright, D., & Brajtman, S. (2011). Relational and embodied knowing: Nursing ethics within the interprofessional team. *Nursing Ethics, 18*(1), 20–30. doi: 10.1177/0969733010386165.

Young, H., Miyamoto, S., Ward, D., Dharmar, M., Yajarayma, T. F., & Berglund, L. (2014). Sustained effects of a nurse coaching intervention via telehealth to improve health behavior change in diabetes. *Telemedicine Journal and E-Health, 20*(9), 828–834.

Zhang, P., Hu, Y. D., Xing, F. M., Li, C. Z., Lan, W. F., & Zhang, X. L. (2017). Effects of a nurse-led transitional care program on clinical outcomes, health-related knowledge, physical and mental health status among Chinese patients with coronary artery disease: A randomized controlled trial. *International Journal of Nursing Studies, 74*(5–6), 34–43.

Appendix A
The Art and Science of Nurse Coaching:
A Provider's Guide to Scope and
Competencies, 1st Edition

The Art & Science of Nurse Coaching

The Provider's Guide to Coaching Scope and Competencies

Darlene R. Hess PhD, RN, AHN-BC, PMHNP-BC, ACC, HWNC-BC
Director, Brown Mountain Visions, Los Ranchos, New Mexico
Faculty, University of Phoenix, Albuquerque, New Mexico
Faculty, Northern New Mexico College, Española, New Mexico
Committee Member, National Consortium for Credentialing of Health and Wellness Coaches

Barbara M. Dossey, PhD, RN, AHN-BC, FAAN, HWNC-BC
Co-Director, International Nurse Coach Association
Core Faculty, Integrative Nurse Coach Certificate Program, Huntington, New York
International Co-Director, Nightingale Initiative for Global Health, Washington, DC and Neepewa, Manitoba, Canada
Director, Holistic Nursing Consultants, Santa Fe, New Mexico
Committee Member, National Consortium for Credentialing of Health and Wellness Coaches

Mary Elaine Southard, MSN, RN, AHN-BC, CHOM, HWNC-BC
Director, Integrative Health Consulting and Coaching, LLC, Scranton, Pennsylvania
Board Member, American Holistic Nurses Credentialing Corporation (AHNCC), Cedar Park, Texas
Committee Member, National Consortium for Credentialing of Health and Wellness Coaches

Susan Luck, MA, RN, HNB-BC, CCN, HWNC-BC
Co-Director, International Nurse Coach Association
Core Faculty, Integrative Nurse Coach Certificate Program, Huntington, New York
Director, EarthRose Institute for Environmental Health, Miami, Florida
Faculty, University of Miami, Clinical Nutrition Program, Department of Family Medicine, Miami, Florida
Committee Member, National Consortium for Credentialing of Health and Wellness Coaches

Bonney Gulino Schaub, MS, RN, PMHCNS-BC, NC-BC
Co-Director, International Nurse Coach Association
Core Faculty, Integrative Nurse Coach Certificate Program
Co-Director and Core Faculty, Huntington Meditation and Imagery Center, Huntington, New York
Committee Member, National Consortium for Credentialing of Health and Wellness Coaches

Linda Bark, PhD, RN, MCC, NC-BC
President, Bark Coaching Institute, Alameda, California
Faculty, JFK Holistic Health Masters Program, Pleasant Hill, California
Faculty/Mentor, National Institute of Whole Health, Boston, Massachusetts
Leadership Team, National Consortium for Credentialing of Health and Wellness Coaches

Silver Spring, Maryland
2013

Appendix A. The Art and Science of Nurse Coaching, 1st Edition

Contents

Appendix A. The Art and Science of Nurse Coaching, 1st Edition

Contributors

Professional Nurse Coaching Workgroup (PNCW) (2009–2012)

Darlene Hess, PhD, AHN-BC, PMHNP-BC, ACC, HWNC-BC, Co-Chair
Barbara M. Dossey, PhD, RN, AHN-BC, FAAN, HWNC-BC, Co-Chair
Mary Elaine Southard, MSN, RN, AHN-BC, CHOM, HWNC-BC
Susan Luck, MA, RN, HNB-BC, CCN, HWNC-BC
Bonney Gulino Schaub, MS, RN, PMHCNS-BC, NC-BC
Linda Bark, PhD, RN, MCC, NC-BC

Professional Nurse Coaching Review Committee (2011–2012)

Phyllis Kritek, PhD, RN, FAAN, Co-Chair
Barbara L. Nichols, DHL, MS, RN, FAAN, Co-Chair
Denys Cope, BSN, RN
Liz Cunningham, MA, RN
Michelle Dart, MSN, RN, CNE
Gail Donner, PhD, RN
Lori Knutson, BSN, RN, HN-BC
Mary Jo Kreitzer, PhD, RN, FAAN
Kristen Lombard, PhD, RN, PMHCNS-BC
Eileen O'Grady, PhD, RN
Diane Pisanos, MS, RN, NNP-E, AHN-BC
Kimberly McNally, MN, RN
Darlene Trandel, PhD, FNP, RN, PCC
Pat Hinton-Walker, PhD, RN, FAAN, CMC, PCC
Mary Wheeler, MEd, RN, PCC
Linda Yoder, PhD, RN, AOCN, FAAN

Appendix A. The Art and Science of Nurse Coaching, 1st Edition

Professional Nurse Coaching Advisory Committee (2011–2012)

Daniel J. Pesut, PhD, RN, PMHCNS-BC, FAAN, Co-Chair
Jean Watson, PhD, RN, FAAN, Co-Chair
Patricia Benner, PhD, RN, FAAN
Nancy Dickerson-Hazard, MSN, RN, CPNP, FAAN
Debra Geradi, MPD, RN, JD
JoEllen Koerner, PhD, RN, FAAN
Mary Jo Kreitzer, PhD, RN, FAAN
Mary Wheeler, MEd, RN, PCC
Beverly Malone, PhD, RN, FAAN
Cheryl A. Peterson, MSN, RN
Franklin A. Shaffer, EdD, RN, FAAN

Endorsing Organizations

The following list is of the endorsing organizations for this document as of December 2012. Other organizations will be added in future editions.

American Academy of Nursing

American Academy of Ambulatory Care Nursing

American Association of Critical Care Nurses

American Holistic Nurses Association

American Holistic Nurses Credentialing Corporation

American Nephrology Nurses Association

American Nurses Association

American Psychiatric Nurses Association

Bark Coaching International

CGFNS International

Emergency Nurses Association

International Association of Human Caring

International Nurse Coach Association

National Gerontological Nursing Association

National League for Nursing

Nurse Organization of Veterans Affairs

Preventive Cardiovascular Nurses Association

Sigma Theta Tau International

Society for the Advancement of Modeling and Role-Modeling

Society of Gastroenterology Nurses and Associates

Watson Caring Science Institute

Preamble

The Art and Science of Nurse Coaching: The Provider's Guide to Coaching Scope and Competencies defines and explains the role of the Nurse Coach within the context of *Nursing: Scope and Standards of Practice*, 2nd Edition (American Nursing Association [ANA], 2010a) and emerging trends in interprofessional health professions education (Interprofessional Education Collaborative Expert Panel, 2011). The International Coach Federation (ICF) Professional Coaching Core Competencies (ICF, 2008a) inform key elements of this document.

The professional Nurse Coach role and coaching are a fundamental part of nursing practice. The professional Nurse Coach role competencies prepare nurses to integrate this role within all specialty areas and settings. Nurse coaching is not a specialty area of nursing practice. Nurse Coaching competencies are based in nursing theories, social and behavioral science theories, and evidence-based promotion of health and well-being. The Nurse Coach uses inquiry and skillfully requests permission to share information instead of coming from an expert role used in patient education and teaching.

Executive Summary

Introduction

There are 3.1 million nurses in the United States (ANA, 2010; American Association of Colleges of Nursing [AACN], 2011) and 17.6 million nurses and midwives in the world (WHO, 2009). The 2010 report from the Institute of Medicine (IOM), *The Future of Nursing* and other health initiatives suggest the need for increased education and leadership from nurses to address the healthcare needs of our nation and world. Nurse Coaches are strategically positioned to skillfully partner with clients to assess, strategize, plan, and evaluate progress towards negotiated coaching goals. Coaching is a natural extension of nursing practice. Professional Nurse Coaches are equipped to implement health-promoting and evidence-based strategies with clients and support behavioral and lifestyle changes to enhance growth, overall health and well-being. With possibilities not yet imagined, employment opportunities for nurses who incorporate coaching into professional practice are developing across the entire spectrum of health, wellness, and healing.

As the healthcare system shifts from a disease-focused and reactive healthcare system to one proactively focused on culturally sensitive wellness, health promotion, and disease prevention, the Nurse Coach role is an essential ingredient of success to assist people towards sustained health. Chronic disease, stress-related illnesses, and entrenched unhealthy lifestyles make health, healing, and well-being challenging to attain and sustain. Nurses need to develop skillful means of partnering and collaborating with clients in new ways, which acknowledge clients as experts in their own care.

Purpose

The purpose of *The Art and Science of Nurse Coaching* is to define and clarify the foundation of the Nurse Coach role and demonstrate nursing's leadership and proactive stance in healthcare transformation.

The Art and Science of Nurse Coaching explains nursing perspectives concerning the role of the Nurse Coach in five key ways: (1) It specifies the philosophy, beliefs, and values of the Nurse Coach and the Nurse Coach's scope of practice; (2) It articulates the relationship between *The Art and Science of Nurse Coaching: The Provider's Guide to Coaching Scope and Competencies* and ANA's *Nursing: Scope and Standards of Practice,* 2nd Edition; (3) It provides the basis for continued interdisciplinary conversations related to professional health and wellness coaches and lay health and wellness coaches; (4) It lays the foundation for an international certification process for professional Nurse Coaching practice; and (5) It identifies the need to develop a core curriculum for professional Nurse Coaching practice that can be used in practice, education, research and the development and evaluation of healthcare policy.

Integrated throughout this document is attention to professional nursing philosophy, values, ethics, and beliefs, an artful use of the nursing process, and contemporary interprofessional collaborative conversations (see the note at the end of this section) related to coaching. The audience for this publication expands beyond nursing proper to include interdisciplinary systems, communities and populations.

Process

The Art and Science of Nurse Coaching delineates the efforts of the Professional Nurse Coach Workgroup (PNCW) (see Contributors section, starting on page vii) and is the product of significant exploratory conversations and electronic mail communication among professional Nurse Coaches and nurse leaders that resulted in a six-step process over a three-year period.

During initial meetings fundamental concepts of Nurse Coaching and the Nurse Coach role as a component of nursing practice were analyzed and discussed. These discussions also included considerations related to the growing emergence of nonprofessional health and wellness coaches as well as the development of health and wellness coaches in other professions. In September 2010, the PNCW circulated *White Paper on Holistic Nurse Coaching* (Hess, Bark, & Southard, 2010) at the National Summit on Standards and Credentialing of Professional Coaches in Healthcare and Wellness (NCCHWC) convened by the National Consortium for the Credentialing of Health and Wellness Coaches in Boston, Massachusetts, to explore the future of health and wellness coaches (NCCHWC, 2010; 2011). *The Art and Science of Nurse Coaching: The Provider's Guide to Coaching Scope and Competencies* has been developed by Nurse Coach experts and vetted via a thorough peer-review process to fully describe the professional Nurse Coach role.

The PNCW entered into a conversation regarding the importance of the role of the Nurse Coach and the need for a national certification process for professional Nurse Coaches with the American Holistic Nurse Credentialing Corporation (AHNCC)(Appendix B). After lengthy discussion, the PNCW entered an agreement with AHNCC whereby AHNCC would sponsor the work of the PNCW in exchange for the rights to establish a national certification process for the Nurse Coach. The PNCW remains engaged in conversations related to alliances with other interprofessional organizations for the purpose of establishing clear guidelines and competencies for professional health and wellness coaches.

An in-depth six-step course of action included the completion of an extensive literature review, compilation of the findings, and development of a draft document. The PNCW engaged with an expert Review Committee and an Advisory Committee comprised of Nurse Coaches and leaders (see Contributors section, starting on page vii). After extensive reviews and several revisions by the PNCW members, the draft document was submitted to the committees for comments, deletions, modifications, and recommendations. Additional reviews were completed and led to the development of a revised document that was sent to the American Nurses Association (ANA) December 1, 2011 to begin the steps towards becoming an endorsed ANA document with additional endorsements from professional nursing organizations.

Definitions and Scope of Practice

[Note: The word client is interchangeable with the word patient throughout this document.]

The Nurse Coach is a registered nurse who integrates coaching competencies into any setting or specialty area of practice to facilitate a process of change or development that assists individuals or groups to realize their potential. Nurse Coaching is a skilled, purposeful, results-oriented, and structured relationship-centered interaction with clients provided by registered nurses for the purpose of promoting achievement of client goals. The Nurse Coach role has roots in Florence Nightingale's legacy, nursing history and theories and the social sciences.

Nurse Coaching involves the ability to develop a coaching partnership, to create a safe space, and to be sensitive to client issues of trust and vulnerability (Schaub & Schaub, 2009) as a basis for further exploration, self-discovery and action planning related to desired outcomes. Coaching builds on client strengths rather than attempting to "fix" weaknesses. The Nurse Coach must be able to explore client readiness for coaching, structure a coaching session, facilitate achievement of the client's desired goals, and co-create a means of determining and evaluating desired outcomes and goals (Hess, Bark, & Southard, 2010). Nurse Coaching is grounded in the principles and core values of professional nursing.

Nurse Coaches are found in all areas of nursing practice and work with individuals and with groups. Nurse Coaches are staff nurses, ambulatory care nurses, case managers, advanced practice nurses, nursing faculty, nurse researchers, educators, administrators, or nurse entrepreneurs. Nurse Coaches may practice in a specialty area such as diabetes education, cardiac rehabilitation, or end-of-life care.

Nurse Coaches may focus on health and wellness coaching, executive coaching, faculty development coaching, managerial coaching, business coaching, or life coaching. The extent to which registered nurses engage in the Nurse Coach role is dependent on coach-specific education, training, experience, position, and the population they serve.

Professional Nurse Coach Competencies and the Nurse Coaching Process

The Art and Science of Nurse Coaching identifies the Nurse Coach competencies that are linked to each of the ANA six standards of practice (assessment, diagnosis, outcomes identification, planning, implementation, evaluation) and ten standards of professional performance (ethics, education, evidence-based practice and research, quality of practice, communication, leadership, collaboration, professional practice evaluation, resources utilization, environmental health) (ANA, 2010a). A description of the professional Nurse Coach role pertaining to each standard is provided followed by the Specific Nurse Coach Competencies related to that standard.

The professional Nurse Coaching competencies are authoritative statements of the duties that all Nurse Coaches are expected to perform competently, regardless of setting or specialization. The list of competencies is not exhaustive. The contents of this document will be expanded as new and broader patterns of the Nurse Coach role are developed and accepted by the nursing profession. The Nurse Coaching competencies are applicable to all areas of Nurse Coaching practice.

The Nurse Coaching Process is a reorientation of the nursing process.

The Nurse Coaching Process includes six steps as follows: (1) Establishing Relationship and Identifying Readiness for Change (Assessment); (2) Identifying Opportunities, Issues, and Concerns (Diagnosis); (3) Establishing Client-Centered Goals (Outcomes); (4) Creating the Structure of the Coaching Interaction (Plan); (5) Empowering and Motivating Clients to Reach Goals (Intervention); and (6) and Assisting Clients to Determine the Extent to which Goals were Achieved (Evaluation).

Summary of Content

The Art and Science of Nurse Coaching is a comprehensive document that further includes a discussion of:

- Foundational professional nursing documents that guide professional Nurse Coaching practice

- Definition of professional Nurse Coach and professional Nurse Coaching practice

- Professional Nurse Coaching scope of practice

- Nurse Coaching process

- Tenets characteristics of professional Nurse Coaching practice

- Healthy environments (internal and external) for professional Nurse Coaching practice

- ANA standards as organizing framework for professional Nurse Coaching practice

- Professional competence in professional Nurse Coaching practice

- Professional Nurse Coaching practice today

- Professional Nurse Coaching research and evidence-based practice

- Progression of curriculum development, certificate programs, and national certification for professional Nurse Coaching

- IOM influences on professional Nurse Coaching practice and leadership

- Integrating the science and art of Nurse Coaching

- Professional trends and issues related to Nurse Coaching

- The Nurse Coach role in national and global healthcare transformation

- Nursing theories and other theories frequently used in professional Nurse Coaching practice

- Interventions frequently used in professional Nurse Coaching practice

- Glossary of terms related to professional Nurse Coaching practice

NOTE

1. In 2010 the National Consortium for the Credentialing of Health and Wellness Coaches (NCCHWC) convened to develop consensus around health and wellness coaching (NCCHWC, 2010; 2011; Wolever & Eisenberg, 2011). Over 80 individuals and organizations representing coaching, health care, and wellness discussed the development of credentialing standards for health and wellness coaching, and the need to integrate coaching skills into the health professions. (See NCCHWC, 2010; 2011). Retrieved from http://www.wellcoaches.com/images/pdf/progressreport-nationalteam-jul-2011.pdf).

Members from the Professional Nurse Coaching Workgroup (PNCW), the American Holistic Nurses Certification Corporation (AHNCC), and the American Holistic Nurses Association (AHNA) attended the meeting. Collaboration continues between the PNCW, nursing and the National Consortium. All PNCW members currently serve on different NCCHWC committees.

Overview of Content

Foundational Professional Nursing Documents That Guide Professional Nurse Coaching Practice

Nurse Coaches are guided in their thinking and decision-making by three professional resources. *Nursing: Scope and Standards of Practice*, 2nd Edition (ANA, 2010a) outlines the expectations of the professional role of registered nurses. It provides the Scope of Practice for all registered nurses and the Standards of Professional Nursing Practice and their accompanying competencies. *Code of Ethics for Nurses with Interpretive Statements* (ANA, 2001) lists the nine provisions that establish the ethical framework for registered nurses across all roles, levels, and settings. *Nursing's Social Policy Statement: The Essence of Professional Practice* (ANA, 2010b) conceptualizes nursing practice, describes the social context of nursing, articulates professional nursing's social contract with society, and provides the definition of nursing.

[Note: The reader is referred to Appendix A for Background, Appendix B for the American Holistic Nurses Credentialing Corporation (AHNCC) Nurse Coach Certification Process, and Appendix C for the Nurse Coach Role in National and Global Healthcare Transformation as related to The Art and Science of Nurse Coaching: The Provider's Guide to Coaching Scope and Competencies.]

Additional Resources

The Art and Science of Nurse Coaching incorporates coaching standards and competencies of the International Coaching Federation (ICF) (2011a). The ICF, with more than 18,000 members in 100 countries (ICF, 2011b), provides independent certification for coaches. ICF certification is a certification process open to all who complete approved coach training, pass an oral and written examination, and meet practice hours requirements. It does not certify any specialties. It does, however, provide a rich resource with an established code of ethics (ICF, 2011c), body of research data, and delineation of practices essential to coaching.

Nurse Coaches practicing in a nursing specialty are also guided by the nursing specialty standards and related documents.

Audience for the Publication

Registered nurses in every role and setting constitute the primary audience of this professional resource. Nurse administrators, organizations and agencies (hospitals, community care centers, long term care facilities) legislators, regulators, legal counsel, and the judiciary system also will benefit from referencing this resource as the dynamic healthcare landscape changes. Those individuals, families, communities, and populations using healthcare and nursing services can use this document to better understand what constitutes professional Nurse Coaching by registered nurses.

Professional Nurse Coach Role: Definition and Scope of Practice

In this section the definition of the professional Nurse Coach role, the contexts of Nurse Coaching, and a detailed description of the practice will be found. In addition are the underlying tenets of practice and the organizing framework based on *Nursing: Scope and Standards of Practice*, 2nd Edition. (ANA, 2010a). *[Note: The word "client" is interchangeable with the word "patient" throughout this document.]*

Definition of Professional Nurse Coach and Professional Nurse Coaching

The professional Nurse Coach is a registered nurse who integrates coaching competencies into any setting or specialty area of practice to facilitate a process of change or development that assists individuals or groups to realize their potential. The change process is grounded in an awareness that effective change evolves from within before it can be manifested and maintained externally. The Nurse Coach works with the whole person, using principles and modalities that integrate body-mind-emotion-spirit-environment.

Professional Nurse Coaching is a skilled, purposeful, results-oriented, and structured relationship-centered interaction with clients provided by registered nurses for the purpose of promoting achievement of client goals. Achievement of client goals is accomplished by first establishing a co-creative partnership with the client where the client is the expert and then by identifying the client's priorities and areas for change. Goals originate from clarifying and identifying the client's agenda.

Professional Nurse Coaching Scope of Practice

The Art and Science of Nurse Coaching describes a competent level of professional Nurse Coaching practice and performance common to all Nurse Coaches. Effective Nurse Coaching interactions involve the ability to develop a coaching partnership, to create a safe space, and to be sensitive to client issues of trust and vulnerability (Schaub & Schaub, 2013; Schaub & Schaub, 2009) as a basis for further exploration, self-discovery and action planning related to desired outcomes. It builds on the client's strengths rather than attempting to "fix" weaknesses. Coaching interactions are based on research findings related to positive psychology (Seligman, 1990; Csikszentmihalyi, 1990) and learned optimism (Seligman, 1990) as it relates to transformational change (Prochaska, et.al., 1995).

The Nurse Coach must be able to explore client readiness for coaching, structure a coaching session, facilitate achievement of the client's desired goals, and co-create a means of determining and evaluating desired outcomes and goals (Hess, Bark, & Southard, 2010). Nurse Coaching is grounded in the principles and core values of professional nursing.

Professional Nurse Coaching practice:

- Incorporates both the *science* (critical thinking, use of evidence/research/ theory [e.g., nursing theories, change theory including appreciative inquiry and motivational interviewing, coherence theory, resilience, complexity science, etc.] and *art* [e.g., intuition, creativity, presence, self-awareness assessment tools and practices, mindfulness, imagery, relaxation, music, etc.]).

- Includes the values and ethics of holism, caring, moral insight, dignity, integrity, competence, responsibility, accountability, and legality that underlie professional nursing.

- Incorporates culturally relevant philosophies and paradigms in a manner that promotes the achievement of client-centered goals.

- Recognizes that coaching interventions, inherent client characteristics, cultural norms, and policies and systems influence client outcomes.

- Honors the relationship between the client's internal and external environment in order to achieve optimal outcomes.

- Partners with the client to identify the client's agenda relative to achievement of the client's goals.

- Creates a safe environment for relationship-centered coaching that includes empathy, warmth, caring, compassion, authenticity, respect, trust, and humor if appropriate.

- Integrates professional nursing and coaching competencies to foster the achievement of client goals.

- Recognizes that self-development (e.g., self-reflection, self-assessment, and self-care) is necessary to provide effective Nurse Coaching services.

- Values self in professional Nurse Coaching practice.

Description and Scope of Professional Nurse Coaching Practice

Nurse Coaches work in all areas of nursing practice and interact with individuals and with groups. Nurse Coaches are staff nurses, ambulatory care nurses, case managers, advanced practice nurses, nursing faculty, nurse researchers, educators, administrators, or nurse entrepreneurs. Nurse Coaches may practice in a specialty area such as diabetes education, cardiac rehabilitation, or end-of-life care.

Nurse Coaches may focus on health and wellness coaching, executive coaching, faculty development coaching, managerial coaching, business coaching, or life coaching. The extent to which registered nurses engage in the Nurse Coach role is dependent on coach specific education, training, experience, position, and the population they serve. The Nurse Coaching competencies are applicable to all areas of professional Nurse Coaching practice.

Development and Function of Professional Nurse Coaching Competencies

The professional Nurse Coaching competencies are authoritative statements of the duties that all Nurse Coaches are expected to perform competently, regardless of setting or specialization. The list of competencies is not exhaustive. The contents of this document will be expanded and revised through time, as new and broader patterns of the Nurse Coach role are developed and accepted by the nursing profession. The Nurse Coach role, scope of practice, tenets, and competencies are subject to formal periodic review and revision.

Application of the competencies is dependent on context. Whether the specifics of each competency apply depends upon the purpose of the coaching interaction. With increased mastery of competencies the nurse is better able to coach the client.

Appendix A. The Art and Science of Nurse Coaching, 1st Edition

The Nursing Process

The nursing process involves six focal areas: assessment, diagnosis, outcomes identification, planning, implementation, and evaluation. These six areas are conceptualized as bi-directional feedback loops from each component (ANA, 2010a). The Nurse Coach uses caring as the essence of professional Nurse Coaching practice (ANA, 2010a) and recognizes the transpersonal dimension of the caring-healing relationship between nurse and client. (Dossey, 2013; Watson, 2007). The Nurse Coach uses the nurse caring process (Potter & Frisch, 2013) with a shift in terminology and meaning to understand and incorporate the client's subjective experience: from *assessment* to establishing a relationship and identifying readiness for change and the resources available to the client for change; from nursing *diagnosis* to identifying opportunities and issues; from *outcomes identification* to having the client set the agenda for achievement of the client's goals; from *planning* to creating the structure of the coaching interaction; from *implementation* to empowering the client to reach goals; and from *evaluation* to assisting the client to determine the extent to which goals were achieved. The Nurse Coach understands that growth and improved health, wholeness, and well-being are the result of an ongoing journey that is ever expanding.

The Nurse Coaching Process

- **Establishing Relationship and Identifying Readiness for Change** (**Assessment**): The Nurse Coach begins by becoming fully present with self and client before initiating the coaching interaction. Cultivating and establishing relationship with the client is a priority for effective coaching. Nurse Coaching is a relationship-centered caring process. Assessment involves identifying the client's strengths, what the client wants to change, and assisting the client to determine his/her readiness for change. Assessment is dynamic and ongoing.

- **Identifying Opportunities, Issues, and Concerns** (**Diagnosis**): The Nurse Coach, in partnership with the client, identifies opportunities and issues related to growth, overall health, wholeness, and well-being. Opportunities for celebrating well-being are explored. The Nurse Coach understands that acknowledgment promotes and reinforces previous successes and serves to enhance further achievements. *Note: There is no attempt or need to assign labels or to establish a diagnosis* *when coaching. Instead the Nurse Coach is open to multiple interpretations of an unfolding interaction.*

- **Establishing Client-Centered Goals (Outcomes identification):** The Nurse Coach employs an overall approach to each coaching interaction that is designed to facilitate achievement of client goals and desired results.

- **Creating the Structure of the Coaching Interaction (Planning):** The Nurse Coach may structure the coaching interaction with a coaching agreement that identifies specific parameters of the coaching relationship, including coach and client responsibilities and action plans.

- **Empowering and Motivating Clients to Reach Goals (Implementation):** The Nurse Coach employs effective communication skills such as deep listening, powerful questioning, and directed dialogue as key components of the coaching interaction. In partnership with the client, the Nurse Coach facilitates learning and results by co-creating awareness, designing actions, setting goals, planning, and addressing progress and accountability. The Nurse Coach skillfully chooses interventions based on the client's statements and actions, and interacts with intention and curiosity in a manner that assists the client toward achievement of the client's goals. The Nurse Coach effectively uses her/his nursing knowledge and a variety of skills acquired with additional coach training.

- **Assisting Client to Determine the Extent to which Goals were Achieved (Evaluation):** The Nurse Coach is aware that evaluation of coaching (the nursing intervention) is done primarily by the client and is based on the client's perception of success and achievement of client-centered goals. The nurse partners with the client to evaluate progress toward goals.

Tenets and Characteristics of Professional Nurse Coaching Practice

The following professional Nurse Coaching tenets are embedded in every competency in this document and are reflected in professional Nurse Coaching practice.

1. The Nurse Coach's practice is individualized for the client.

The Nurse Coach encourages growth, wholeness, and well-being of the client according to the client's values and beliefs, and believes that every client is creative, resourceful, and whole. A *client* is defined as the person, patient, family member, community, group, or population. There is unity, totality, and connectedness of everyone and everything: human beings are unique and inherently good. People are able to find meaning and purpose in life experiences. All people have an innate power and capacity for the achievement of well-being. People are the recipients of Nurse Coaching services.

2. The Nurse Coach establishes a coaching relationship with the client.

The Nurse Coach establishes a coaching relationship as foundational to the success of a coaching interaction. It is a relationship where the complexity of human experiences is valued. The Nurse Coach demonstrates unconditional positive regard for clients and accepts them where they are. Within the Nurse Coach–client relationship, it is understood that change is best achieved when aligned with the client's goals and desires and readiness for change.

3. Human caring is central to professional Nurse Coaching practice.

Human caring is the moral ideal of nursing in which the nurse brings one's entire self into a relationship with the whole self of the client in order to protect the client's vulnerability, preserve her or his humanity and dignity, and reinforce the meaning and experience of oneness and unity.

4. The Nurse Coach uses the Nurse Coaching process to guide nurse-client coaching interactions.

The Nurse Coaching process is a systematic and skilled process that incorporates approaches to nursing practice and the coaching process that are holistic, integrative, and integral. The nursing process is expanded and reinterpreted to include widely used nursing theories and evidence-based behavioral change theories and frameworks that redefine established concepts and terms. The Nurse Coach understands and adheres to professional and ethical standards that include providing respectful, compassionate, and culturally relevant integrative nursing care to all persons.

5. **The Nurse Coach recognizes the link between the internal and external environment of self and the client.**

Each component influences growth, health, optimal functioning, and well-being.

Healthy Environments (Internal and External) for Professional Nurse Coaching Practice

The environment is the context within which all living systems participate and interact, including the physical body and its habitat along with cultural, psychological, social, and historical influences. It includes both the external physical space and the person's internal physical, mental, emotional, social, and spiritual experience. Well-being is possible for all. Illness and/or imbalance provide opportunities for learning and movement toward change to enhance well-being (AHNA/ANA, 2013).

ANA Standards as Organizing Framework for Professional Nurse Coaching Practice

The six Standards of Practice and ten Standards of Professional Performance in *Nursing: Scope and Standards of Practice,* 2nd Edition (ANA, 2010a) provide the organizing framework for *The Art and Science of Nurse Coaching.* Competencies specific to the professional Nurse Coach role that are described in this document (starting on page 27) are linked to those standards, which are reproduced in the following table for the convenience of the reader.

Standards of Practice	Standards of Professional Practice
The Standards of Practice describe a competent level of nursing care as demonstrated by the critical thinking model known as the nursing process. The nursing process includes the components of assessment, diagnosis, outcomes identification, planning, implementation, and evaluation. Accordingly, the nursing process encompasses significant actions taken by registered nurses and forms the foundation of the nurse's decision-making.	The Standards of Professional Performance describe a competent level of behavior in the professional role, including activities related to ethics, education, evidence-based practice and research, quality of practice, communication, leadership, collaboration, professional practice evaluation, resource utilization, and environmental health.
Standard 1. Assessment The registered nurse collects comprehensive data pertinent to the healthcare consumer's health and/or the situation.	All registered nurses are expected to engage in professional role activities, including leadership, appropriate to their education and position. Registered nurses are accountable for their professional actions to themselves, their healthcare consumers, their peers, and ultimately to society.
Standard 2. Diagnosis The registered nurse analyzes the assessment data to determine the diagnoses or the issues.	**Standard 7. Ethics** The registered nurse practices ethically.
Standard 3. Outcomes Identification The registered nurse identifies expected outcomes for a plan individualized to the healthcare consumer or the situation.	**Standard 8. Education** The registered nurse attains knowledge and competence that reflects current nursing practice.
Standard 4. Planning The registered nurse develops a plan that prescribes strategies and alternatives to attain expected outcomes.	**Standard 9. Evidence-Based Practice and Research** The registered nurse integrates evidence and research findings into practice.
Standard 5. Implementation The registered nurse implements the identified plan.	**Standard 10. Quality of Practice** The registered nurse contributes to quality nursing practice.
Standard 6. Evaluation The registered nurse evaluates progress toward attainment of outcomes.	**Standard 11. Communication** The registered nurse communicates effectively in a variety of formats in all areas of practice.
	Standard 12. Leadership The registered nurse demonstrates leadership in the professional practice setting and the profession.
	Standard 13. Collaboration The registered nurse collaborates with healthcare consumer, family, and others in the conduct of nursing practice.

Standards of Practice	Standards of Professional Practice
	Standard 14. Professional Practice Evaluation The registered nurse evaluates her or his own nursing practice in relation to professional practice standards and guidelines, relevant statutes, and regulations.
	Standard 15. Resource Utilization The registered nurse utilizes appropriate resources to plan and provide nursing services that are safe, effective, and financially responsible.
	Standard 16. Environmental Health The registered nurse practices in an environmentally safe and healthy manner.

Professional Competence in Nurse Coaching Practice

Professional Nurse Coaching competence can be taught, defined, measured, and evaluated. There is no single method of evaluation or tool that can guarantee competence. Competence is dynamic and situational and is recognized as an ongoing process resulting in appropriate outcome/s. The context of a coaching relationship/coaching interaction determines what competencies are necessary. Assurance of competence is the shared responsibility of individual nurses, professional nursing organizations, credentialing and certification entities, and other key stakeholders.

Definitions and Concepts Related to Professional Nurse Coaching Competence

The following ideas are central to the discussion of Nurse Coaching competence:

- A Nurse Coach who demonstrates competence (per the competencies in this document) is performing at an expected level.

- A Nurse Coach competency is an expected level of performance that

Appendix A. The Art and Science of Nurse Coaching, 1st Edition

integrates knowledge, skills, abilities, and judgment.

- A Nurse Coach integrates knowledge, skills, abilities, and judgment in formal, informal, and reflective learning experiences.
- A Nurse Coach has integrity.
- A Nurse Coach is aware of her/his own strengths and weaknesses, has positive self-regard, and is open to feedback.
- A Nurse Coach values and uses intuitive knowing.
- Nurse Coaching involves emotional, moral, and spiritual intelligence.
- Nurse Coaching demonstrates an understanding of science and humanities, professional standards of practice, coaching competencies, insights gained from experiences, personal strengths, resources, and capabilities, and leadership performance.
- Nurse Coaching includes psychomotor, communication, interpersonal, and environmental skills.
- Nurse Coaching judgment includes critical thinking, problem-solving, ethical reasoning, decision-making, and clinical leadership.
- Nurse Coach learning may occur in academic settings, professional practice environments, structured certificate programs, and online educational offerings.
- Nurse Coach reflective learning is recurrent thoughtful self-assessment, analysis, and synthesis of strengths and opportunities for improvement.

Competence and Competency in Professional Nurse Coaching Practice

The competent Nurse Coach considers the person, family, and/or group being coached and the setting and available resources. The Nurse Coach considers factors that either enhance or detract from the ability to conduct a coaching session or coaching interaction. The Nurse Coach addresses barriers that constrain competent practice. The ability to perform at the expected level requires lifelong learning and self-development (self-reflection, self-assessment, self-evaluation, and self-care). Nurse Coaches continually assess and reassess their competencies and identify areas where new knowledge, skills, integral learning experiences, and self-development can enhance personal and professional self-development.

Evaluating Competence

Competence is evaluated using measurement tools that capture qualitative and quantitative data about the Nurse Coach's basic knowledge and performance. However, no single tool or method can guarantee competence.

Professional Nurse Coaching Practice Today

Statistical Snapshot

There are 3.1 million nurses in the United States (ANA, 2010a; AACN, 2011). It is the largest segment of the nation's healthcare workforce. A major shift is underway in the United States to move from a disease-based model of care to a health and wellness promotion model. New national prevention strategies are being considered and implemented. Currently there are 17.6 millions nurses and midwives engaged in providing healthcare around the world (WHO, 2009).

The role of the Nurse Coach is fundamental to professional nursing (Schaub, Luck & Dossey, 2013). The Nurse Coach role has roots in social sciences, holism, and nursing theory. Nurse coaching competencies are based in nursing, behavioral science, and health promotion theories and research. Development of professional Nurse Coaching skills, which integrate basic coaching skills with the unique dimensions that shape nursing practice, is not typically included in the curriculums of nursing educational programs. The focused preparation of Nurse Coaches is integral to ensuring these services are available to patients.

Health and wellness coaches without a professional health background have emerged. In 2010 the National Consortium for the Credentialing of Health and Wellness Coaches (NCCHWC) convened to develop consensus around health and wellness coaching (National Consortium for the Credentialing of Health and Wellness Coaches Progress Report July, 2011; Wolever & Eisenberg, 2011). Over 80 individuals and organizations representing coaching, health care, and wellness discussed the development of credentialing standards for health and wellness coaching, and the need to integrate coaching competencies into the health professions.

It is an important time for the nursing profession to expand its visibility by embracing the professional Nurse Coach role and the emerging coaching paradigm. With the national focus on prevention and wellness promotion, it is essential for nursing to have an increased presence in health and wellness efforts designed to improve health outcomes and reduce health costs for individuals, employers, insurance companies, and the nation.

Nurse Coaches must assume a significant leadership role in these efforts. It is critical that available professional nurse resources be maximized to reduce the prevalence and severity of chronic illness. Nurse Coaches are equipped to implement health-promoting strategies with clients, supporting behavioral and lifestyle changes to enhance growth, overall health and well-being.

The Art and Science of Nurse Coaching describes the role of the Nurse Coach. It will assist nurses as they assume the position of Nurse Coach in hospitals, clinics, communities, and in private professional nurse practices. It will serve as a guide in the development of Nurse Coach educational programs. Reimbursement is also needed for Nurse Coaching that is already being provided in wellness promotion programs that are included within managed care contracts that have been implemented into new Medicare programs.

Roots of Professional Nurse Coaching

Florence Nightingale (1820–1910)—the foundational philosopher of modern nursing—established nursing practice that could be measured by evaluating outcomes. She advocated, identified, and focused on factors that promote health recognized today as environmental and social determinants of health—the same factors that Nurse Coaches now promote to achieve optimal health and well-being (Dossey, 2013; Dossey, 2010; Dossey, Selanders, Beck, & Attewell, 2005; Nightingale, 1859, 1860, 1893). Nightingale emphasized the necessity for nursing to be a profession, and that nurses must be educated, and not "trained." She established the imperative of evidence-based practice, a nursing standard now widely known to be as important as she had known it to be. Nightingale was the first recognized nurse theorist—a clinical educator, scientist, statistician, environmentalist, policy maker, social activist, facilitator, communicator, and visionary. Her contributions to nursing theory, research, statistics, public health, healthcare reform, and Nurse Coaching are foundational and inspirational. In 1893 Nightingale wrote:

..."In the future which I shall not see, for I am old, may a better way be opened! May the methods by which every infant, every human being will have the best chance at health—the methods by which every sick person will have the best chance at recovery, be learned and practiced. Hospitals are only an intermediate stage of civilization, never intended, at all events, to take in the whole sick population.

May we hope that, when we are all dead and gone, leaders will arise who have been personally experienced in the hard, practical work, the difficulties, and the joys of organizing nursing reforms, and who will lead far beyond anything we have done..."

Nightingale left 21st-century nurses with a call. Nurse Coaches bring an integrative, holistic perspective to coaching (Dossey, 2013; Dossey, 2010; Hess et al., 2010). Nurse theorists and scholars have created models for working with the whole person that incorporate the biological, psychological, social/cultural, environmental, and transpersonal and energetic components of individuals. Integral perspectives allow for openness and "not knowing" (Dossey, 2009) – a way to where new knowledge resides. Erickson views this broad outlook as "integrative knowing," "a way to bring together "multiple ways-of-knowing, integrating and creating new knowledge" (Erickson, 2010, p. 65). Some Nurse Coaches utilize a holistic, integral model of coaching as a way to frame coaching interactions (Bark, 2011; Bark Coaching Institute, n.d.; Integrative Nurse Coach Certificate Program, n.d.).

Professional Nurse Coaching Research and Evidence-Based Practice

Professional Nurse Coaching research is relevant to learning, documenting, and comprehending the science and art of Nurse Coaching. To increase the understanding of professional Nurse Coaching practice and to enhance the evidence-base, research may include descriptive, explanatory and exploratory designs. This may be accomplished by using qualitative, quantitative, mixed methods or other approaches. Professional Nurse Coaching research is needed to further the understanding of the Nurse Coach–client relationship. This will support identifying the factors that contribute to increased client efficacy and ability to successfully achieve the changes that enhance life satisfaction, growth, health, and well-being.

Evidence-based practice is the conscientious use of the best available evidence combined with clinician's expertise and judgment, and patient's preferences and values to arrive at the best decisions leading to quality outcomes (Baldwin, Schultz, Melynk, & Rycoft-Malone, 2013). Nurse Coaches honor the individual's subjective health experiences, health beliefs, and values. Nurse Coaches develop therapeutic partnerships with individuals, families, and communities that are grounded in nursing knowledge, theories, research expertise, intuition, and creativity. Nurse researchers are encouraged to design Nurse Coaching research studies that incorporate theories, conceptual frameworks, and a paradigm that strengthens the understanding of the whole person (Zahourek, 2013.)

Professional Nurse Coaching research and evidence-based practice is growing. Numerous articles in scholarly nursing journals referring to Nurse Coaching have been published (Hess & Dossey, in press). As the national focus continues to move from disease care to health promotion and wellness, additional research is needed.

Professional Nurse Coaching in Advocacy and Society

Chronic disease and stress related illnesses are increasing. The fast pace of daily life, lack of exercise, poor food choices, and environmental risk factors are frequently implicated. Nurse Coaching is critical to assisting individuals, families, and groups to make the changes that foster self-awareness and promote healthier lifestyles.

Nurse Coaches have the skills and knowledge to empower individuals to make beneficial changes. Furthermore, Nurse Coaches have the ability to help transform the health of our nation and our world as they engage in interprofessional conversations and partnerships to facilitate the changes that lead to improved health and well-being.

Progression of Professional Nurse Coaching Curriculum Development, Nurse Coaching Certificate Programs, and Professional Nurse Coaching Certification

As the role of the Nurse Coach has evolved, it is apparent that the term *coach* is loosely defined and often confused with the role of preceptor, mentor, counselor, navigator, or educator. Although growing in popularity, the role of the Nurse Coach has not been clearly defined. *The Art and Science of Nurse Coaching* addresses the need to clearly define the role of the Nurse Coach and provides a guide for nurses across all nursing specialties, for Nurse Coach curriculum development, for Nurse Coach certificate programs, and for Nurse Coach certification.

Health and wellness programs, health maintenance organizations, health insurance companies, and agencies that provide case management services are increasingly employing nurses as coaches to assist individuals in achieving improved health outcomes. Many nurses in hospitals and community agencies have added coaching skills to their nursing practice as a new strategy or intervention to assist patients. Some nurses who professionally pursue such coaching have created successful and thriving businesses providing coach training and coaching services to private clients, groups, and organizations. These early indicators of the importance and impact of nurses as professional coaches emphasize the urgency in formally defining the role, scope of practice, and competencies of the Nurse Coach.

In the 1950s, nursing theorists Hildegard Peplau and Dorothea Orem introduced several concepts and practices that are now seen as important elements of professional Nurse Coaching practice.

Peplau (1952) described the nurse's task as recognizing and mobilizing the person's innate capacity for self-healing and growth. Her perspective originated in a belief that every individual is a unique being with the capacity to learn, develop, and change. She saw the role of the nurse as collaborating and partnering with the client to establish a relationship that would assist the client to realize these potentials. She wrote of the importance of the nurse's self-awareness and self-knowledge in order that this process would occur free of the nurse's needs and agendas. Peplau wrote of clarifying, listening, accepting and interpreting what the client shared in the interpersonal relationship. As part of the resolution process, the nurse would assist the client in establishing new goals, if desired.

Orem (1971) first wrote of her self-care model of nursing in 1953. Her work emerged from a philosophy of health as a state of wholeness. She identified self-care as a key element in maintaining human structure and functioning throughout the lifecycle. The nurse works with clients in helping to identify their self-care deficits. The nurse then helps the client to overcome the deficits by addressing the client's capacity and motivation to do so. Orem recognized that taking responsibility for self-care was a role change for the client. She wrote of the importance of the client-nurse relationship as being instrumental in supporting a process of change.

Patricia Benner (1985), the prominent nurse leader, theorist, and author of the nursing textbook *From Novice to Expert* (Benner, 1984) used the term *nurse coach* nearly 30 years ago to describe the patient–nurse partnership and a conceptual framework based on social support theory. In her model, the nurse responds to and interacts with the client to create joint decision-making regarding goals and methods to achieve goals. This coaching or partnering process involves a nursing perspective that includes holism and self-care and guides Nurse Coaches in the mobilization of inner resources and inner wisdom.

Schenk (2002) described the nurse coach as a healthcare resource for this millennium. Southard (2003) developed a health coach integrative model of care for nurses with accompanying standards of practice based on the core values of holistic nursing. Hayes and Kalmakis (2007) described coaching as a significant strategy available to nurse practitioners to promote health and wellness by inviting the active participation of the individual receiving healthcare services. In 2008 Watson developed the Caring Science Caritas Coaching Education Program (CCEP) (Watson Caring Science Institute, n.d.). Watson's Caritas Coaching Program focuses on intelligent heart-centered approaches to health care by translating and sustaining the ethic, philosophy, theory, and practice of the Science of Human Caring into systems and society (Watson Caring Science Institute, n.d.).

In 2009, the International Council of Nurses (ICN), a federation of more than 130 national nursing organization and representing millions of nurses worldwide, partnered with the Honor Society of Nursing, Sigma Theta Tau International (STTI), representing over 125,000 nurses worldwide, and published *Coaching in Nursing* (Donner & Wheeler, 2009) to support this direction for professional development of nurses.

McNally and Cunningham (2010) developed a coaching model that focuses on helping nurse leaders conduct coaching conversations for development of coaching cultures in the workplace. Bark (2011) developed an integral model of coaching based on structures of consciousness and integral theory that has been taught and used by many nurses in professional nursing practice. Bark's coaching model provides a multidimensional foundation and methods for coaching and coach training (Bark Coaching Institute, n.d.). Dossey, Luck, and Schaub developed the Integrative Nurse Coach Certificate Program (INCCP) based on integral theory, the vulnerability model, and the integrative functional health model, as well as other recognized coaching theories and competencies. Nurses develop coaching skills to assist clients in the achievement of health and wellness goals and to navigate the complex world of medical care (Integrative Nurse Coach Certificate Program, n.d.).

IOM Influences on Professional Nurse Coaching Practice and Leadership

Undertaking a two-year study started in 2008, the Robert Wood Johnson Foundation (RWJF) and the Institute of Medicine (IOM) partnered to assess the future of the nursing profession. The intention was to determine ways to transform the profession of nursing. The outcome of this process was a report that makes recommendations for an action-oriented blueprint for the future of nursing.

The IOM report *The Future of Nursing* (2010) developed four key messages:

- Nurses should practice to the full extent of their education and training.

- Nurses should achieve higher levels of education and training through an improved education system that promotes seamless academic progression.

- Nurses should be full partners, with physicians and other healthcare professionals, in redesigning health care in the United States.

- Effective workforce planning and policy making require better data collection and information infrastructure.

As the United States transforms its healthcare system, professional Nurse Coaches are emerging as leaders who play a fundamental role in informing the government, regulatory agencies, businesses, and organizations about professional Nurse Coaching practice.

Integrating the Science and Art of Nurse Coaching

Nurse Coaching Core Values

Nurse Coaches understand that the professional Nurse Coach role, scope of practice, and competencies are linked to each of the ANA six Standards of Practice and ten Standards of Professional Performance (ANA, 2010a). The professional Nurse Coach role is based upon the following five core values: (1) Nurse Coach Philosophy, Theories, Ethics; (2) Nurse Coaching Process; (3) Nurse Coach Communication, Coaching Environment; (4) Nurse Coach Education, Research, Leadership; and (5) Nurse Coach Self-Development (Self-Reflection, Self-Assessment, Self-Evaluation, Self-Care).

Appendix A. The Art and Science of Nurse Coaching, 1st Edition

These core values and the specific Nurse Coaching competencies—which are aligned with *Nursing: Scope and Standards of Practice*, 2nd Edition (ANA, 2010a) and *Holistic Nursing: Scope and Standards*, 2nd Edition. (AHNA & ANA, 2013)—are the foundation for curriculum development, while *Professional Nurse Coach Core Curriculum* (Dossey & Hess, in press), and the nationally recognized American Holistic Nurses Credentialing Corporation (AHNCC) Nurse Coach Certification process (see Appendix B). Nurse Coaches understand that professional Nurse Coaching practice is defined by these core values and competencies. Nurse Coaching enhances foundational professional nursing skills that are acquired by additional training.

The Science of Nurse Coaching

Nurse Coaches incorporate approaches to nursing practice that are holistic, integrative, and integral and which include the work of numerous nurse scholars. Nurse Coaching is a systematic and skilled process grounded in scholarly evidenced-based professional nursing practice. (Appendix C discusses nursing and other related theories and concepts commonly utilized in professional Nurse Coaching practice.)

The Art of Nurse Coaching

The nurse caring process guides the establishment of core values and competencies of professional Nurse Coaching practice, whether used with individuals, families, groups, or communities. At the heart of Nurse Coaching is growth of the body-mind-spirit system on various levels. The quality of human caring is central in the Nurse Coach–client relationship. The nurse brings her/his self into the coaching relationship with the whole self of the patient/client. This relationship provides the client with a safe environment in which to express their feelings, goals, hopes, dreams, and share their vulnerability, pain, and suffering.

This relationship allows a flow of energy in the body-mind-spirit system of each that may be manifested as creativity, coherence, resilience, or anxiety, fear and frustration (Koerner, 2011). The Nurse Coach holds the container for what needs to be expressed. In the coaching relationship there may be various shifts in consciousness, intrapersonal dynamics, interpersonal relationships, and expressions of the lived experiences of connection, unity, and oneness with the larger environment, cosmos, or Spirit, however defined. Ideally Nurse Coaches embody the following qualities (Dossey, Luck, & Schaub, 2013):

- Development of integrative, integral, and holistic perspectives that include a bio-psycho-social-spiritual-cultural-environmental model of the person

- Recognition that self-healing is an on-going process and necessitates intentionality

- Willingness to model self-development (self-reflection, self-assessments, self-evaluation, self-care)

- Willingness to identify creative and self-defeating patterns in self

- Willingness to take responsibility for inner reactions to clients and situations

- Commitment to maintain a sense of presence, authenticity, and self-awareness in nursing practice

- Cultivation of a capacity for deep listening, mindful presence, and not-knowing

- Respect and love for the humanness of clients

- Commitment to creativity and innovation

- Willingness to bear witness to a client's pain and suffering

- Willingness to believe that change is possible for all

- Commitment to life-long personal self-development and learning

In professional Nurse Coaching practice the nurse attends to the client's subjective experiences and the client's internal frame of reference. The Nurse Coach views clients as resourceful individuals with inherent answers and wisdom. The client chooses the topics for coaching and determines the direction of the coaching session. The nurse sets aside the expert role. There is no predetermined information or education to be offered, and there are no predetermined objectives or outcomes identified.

Professional Nurse Coaching recognizes and supports the client's current way of being as the client evolves towards desired changes and goals. The Nurse Coach spends time with the client in discovery and only moves into the nurse expert role, when indicated, to assist the client. The Nurse Coach remembers that "less is more" when it comes to teaching or advising. What needs to be shared emerges as the nurse "walks with the client" through the discovery process.

The Nurse Coach is present, curious, attentive to the present moment, and thus open to what emerges, free of any predetermined idea of what needs to be "fixed" in the client. The Nurse Coach listens carefully and attentively to the thread of a client's story, perspectives, and reality while engaging in a skillful and free-flowing process of discovery. The Nurse Coach trusts her/his intuition regarding what to say next, and is not thinking about the next question. By skillfully using the "power of the pause," the Nurse Coach communicates being comfortable with silence and is then able to be totally present and open to what the client is expressing.

Professional Nurse Coaching Societal and Ethical Dimensions

Nurses are bound by a professional code of ethics (ANA, 2001). At the heart of nursing's social contract with society is self-regulation by the nursing profession that assures quality performance. Nurses are responsive to the changing needs of society regarding the expansion of theoretical and scientific parameters related to human flourishing, health promotion and disease prevention. Nurse Coaches are accountable for their performance. They engage in quality reviews to further refine their professional knowledge, competence, communication, and leadership.

Nurse Coaches work independently as well as collaboratively to leverage overlapping skills that complement individual efforts (ANA, 2010a). Recognizing the expertise of interprofessional colleagues, they make referrals when appropriate. This may entail shared responsibilities with a common focus on clients' reaching their highest potential. Nurse Coaches recognize their constantly changing professional practice boundaries. Nurse Coaches frequently evaluate safety, effectiveness, and costs related to the services they provide. They are committed to lifelong learning.

Caring and Professional Nurse Coach Practice

Caring is the essence of nursing and central to the professional Nurse Coach role. Human caring is the moral ideal of nursing in which the nurse brings one's entire self into a relationship with the whole self of the client in order to protect the client's vulnerability, preserve her or his humanity and dignity, and reinforce the meaning and experience of oneness and unity. Nurse Coaches recognize the transpersonal caring-healing process (Dossey, 2013; Watson,

2007) that involves temporarily transcending or moving beyond one's usual identification with the limited biological, historical, cultural, and personal self; this occurs at the deepest and most profound levels of human experience possible. Transpersonal refers to that which transcends the limits and boundaries of individual ego identities and possibilities to include acknowledgment and appreciation of something greater.

Continued Commitment to Professional Nurse Coaching

Nurse Coaches remain involved in continuous learning and self-development to enhance Nurse Coaching practice. Nurse Coaches may demonstrate commitment to their practices by their involvement in professional associations and community organizations, by acquiring additional education, or by other self-development activities (e.g. supervision, continuing education, reflection, self-assessment, lifestyle changes).

Nurse Coaches possess the knowledge, skills, and abilities to assist clients to achieve goals. Nurse Coaches facilitate changes that foster improved health and well-being for all regardless of cultural background, value system, religious belief, gender, sexual identity, or disability. Nurse Coaches believe that change is possible and are willing to hold that vision for all.

Professional Trends and Issues Related to Professional Nurse Coaching

It is estimated that 270 billion dollars a year is spent on disease management— on attempting to cure acute disease and treat chronic disease. According to the Centers for Disease Control and Prevention, in 2009, approximately 133 million Americans—nearly 1 in 2 adults—were living with at least one chronic illness and more than 70% of healthcare costs were due to preventable lifestyle-related diseases (Snyderman & Dinan, 2010). Currently, with eight out of ten people over 25 years of age overweight, and with childhood obesity spiraling out of control, the future burden on our health system and society provides an imperative to seek new directions to halt these trends (Luck, 2010). It is estimated that over ten years, $900 billion can be saved with lifestyle medicine (Hyman, Ornish, & Roizen, 2010). Lifestyle medicine involves engaging individuals in health promotion, assisting them to be proactive, participatory, and to partner with healthcare providers and others in creating new and sustainable health behaviors.

Chronic disease is now seen as a global epidemic and a driver for rising healthcare costs. The World Health Organization (WHO, 2011) reports that cardiovascular diseases (heart disease and strokes), cancers, diabetes and chronic lung disease are today the leading causes of disease burden and death worldwide. The four major causative chronic disease risk factors are tobacco use, unhealthy diet, lack of physical activity, and the harmful use of alcohol. Chronic illness is seen as a cause for early mortality that has now surpassed communicable disease.

The Patient Protection and Affordable Care Act, the Healthy People 2020 Initiative, and the National Prevention Strategy (see more below) have increased the national conversations related to new healthcare strategies.

Patient Protection and Affordable Care Act

On March 23, 2010, the Patient Protection and Affordable Care Act (PPACA) became law (HR3590) (The Patient Protection and Affordable Care Act, 2010). The language in the PPACA refers to partnerships in Section 4001 includes partnerships with a diverse group of licensed health professionals including practitioners of integrative health, preventive medicine, health coaching, public education, and more.

Healthy People 2020 Initiative

In December 2010 the Healthy People 2020 initiative (U.S. Department of Health and Human Services, n.d.) was announced. This initiative continues the work started in 2000 with the Healthy People 2010 initiative for improving the nation's health. The Healthy People 2020 initiative is the result of a multiyear process that reflects input from a diverse group of individuals and organizations. The leading health indicators are increased physical activity, overweight and obesity, tobacco use, substance abuse, responsible healthy sexual behavior, mental health, injury and violence, environmental quality, immunization, and access to health care. These health indicators were selected on the basis of their ability to motivate action, the availability of data to measure progress, and their importance as public health issues.

The vision, mission, and overarching goals provide structure and guidance for achieving the Healthy People 2020 objectives. While general in nature, they offer specific, important areas of emphasis where action must be taken if the United States is to achieve better health by the year 2020. Developed under the leadership of the Federal Interagency Workgroup (FIW), the Healthy People

2020 framework is the product of an exhaustive collaborative process among the U.S. Department of Health and Human Services (HHS) and other federal agencies, public stakeholders, and the advisory committee.

The Healthy People 2020 mission is to:

- Identify nationwide health improvement priorities.

- Increase public awareness and understanding of the determinants of health, disease, and disability and the opportunities for progress.

- Provide measurable objectives and goals that are applicable at the national, State, and local levels.

- Engage multiple sectors to take actions to strengthen policies and improve practices that are driven by the best available evidence and knowledge.

- Identify critical research, evaluation, and data collection needs.

The overall goals of Healthy People 2020 are to:

- Attain high-quality, longer lives free of preventable disease, disability, injury, and premature death.

- Achieve health equity, eliminate disparities, and improve the health of all groups.

- Create social and physical environments that promote good health for all.

- Promote quality of life, healthy development, and healthy behaviors across all life stages.

National Prevention Strategy

On June 16, 2011, the National Prevention, Health Promotion, and Public Health Council, including Surgeon General Regina Benjamin, MD, Department of Health and Human Services (HHS) Secretary Kathleen Sebelius, and others announced the release of the National Prevention and Health Promotion Strategy. Referred to subsequently as the National Prevention Strategy, it is a comprehensive plan that will help increase the number of Americans who are healthy at every stage of life (National Prevention Council, 2011, 2012). To stop disease before it starts and to create strategies for a healthy and fit nation, prevention must become part of daily life. The National Prevention Strategy recognizes that good health comes not just from receiving quality medical care, but also from clean air and water, safe worksites and healthy foods. The strategy was created through the PPACA and developed by the National Prevention Council, which is comprised of the heads of 17 Federal agencies that consulted with outside experts and stakeholders.

The National Prevention Strategy includes actions that public and private partners can take to help Americans stay healthy and fit and improve our nation's prosperity. The strategy outlines four strategic directions that, together, are fundamental to improving the nation's health:

- Building Healthy and Safe Community Environments: Prevention of disease starts in our communities and at home; not just in the doctor's office.

- Expanding Quality Preventive Services in Both Clinical and Community Settings: When people receive preventive care, such as immunizations and cancer screenings, they have better health and lower healthcare costs.

- Empowering People to Make Healthy Choices: When people have access to actionable and easy-to-understand information and resources, they are empowered to make healthier choices.

- Eliminating Health Disparities: By eliminating disparities in achieving and maintaining health, we can help improve quality of life for all Americans.

Other Federal Health and Wellness Programs

Specific actions are underway by the Obama Administration to implement programs to improve Americans' lives, including the America's Great Outdoors Initiative, the Neighborhood Revitalization Initiative, and Executive Order 13548 to make the federal government a model employer of persons with disabilities. Through these and other programs, the Obama Administration is working to ensure every American has the opportunity to live the healthiest life possible.

Nurse Coaches will be of assistance in achieving the goals of the Patient Protection and Affordable Care Act, the Healthy People 2020 Initiative, the National Prevention Strategy, and other programs being implemented to improve health and well-being for all.

Summary of the Scope of Nurse Coaching Practice

With a renewed focus on prevention and wellness promotion in healthcare reform, now is an important time for the nursing profession to expand its visibility in the emerging coaching paradigm. As various strategies gain momentum for the training of wellness coaches, Nurse Coaches are uniquely positioned to coach and engage individuals in the process of behavior change.

Professional Nurse Coach Practice and Performance Competencies

Professional Nurse Coach competencies are linked to each of the ANA six Standards of Practice and ten Standards of Professional Performance (ANA, 2010a). A description of the professional Nurse Coach role pertaining to each standard is provided followed by the specific Nurse Coach competencies related to that standard.

[Note: Professional Nurse Coach practice competencies include the ICF competencies.]

Professional Nurse Coach Practice Competencies

ANA Standard 1. Assessment
The registered nurse collects comprehensive data pertinent to the healthcare consumer's health and/or the situation.

Professional Nurse Coach Role
Setting the foundation for coaching begins during the assessment phase of the coaching interaction. Assessment begins by becoming fully present with self and client before initiating the coaching interaction. Assessment proceeds to establishing a relationship with the client and access to the client's subjective experience/story and internal frame of reference through the cultivation and establishment of a relationship. The Nurse Coach determines if the client's concerns are appropriate for the coaching role. The Nurse Coach helps the client assess readiness and available resources for change. Assessment is dynamic and ongoing.

Appendix A. The Art and Science of Nurse Coaching, 1st Edition

Professional Nurse Coach Competencies

The Nurse Coach:

1. Becomes fully present to self and client prior to collecting data pertinent to the coaching interaction.

2. Co-creates a relationship between the Nurse Coach and the client that promotes trust and intimacy.

3. Recognizes and respects the client as the authority on her or his own health and well-being.

4. Explores with the client why coaching is being considered at this time and what the client wants to address during the coaching interaction.

5. Ensures that the client sets the agenda for the coaching session and holds the client's agenda throughout the session.

6. Helps the client assess stage of readiness for change (pre-contemplation, contemplation, preparation, action, maintenance).

7. Incorporates various types of knowing, including intuition, and validates this intuitive knowledge with the client when appropriate.

8. Explores, through powerful questions and feedback, multiple sources of information to assist the client to become aware of areas for coaching.

9. Uses appropriate evidence-informed whole person assessment techniques and instruments, with the client's permission, and with appropriate training.

10. Determines the need for, and refers the client to, other professionals and services as appropriate.

11. Assesses if there is an effective working match between the coach and the prospective client.

12. Understands and effectively discusses with the client the ethical guidelines and specific parameters of the Nurse Coaching relationship (e.g., logistics, fees, scheduling).

13. Co-creates with the client an agreement that identifies the role of the Nurse Coach and the role of the client.

ANA Standard 2. Diagnosis

The registered nurse analyzes the assessment data to determine the diagnoses or the issues.

Professional Nurse Coach Role

The Nurse Coach and the client together explore assessment data to determine areas for change.

Professional Nurse Coach Competencies

The Nurse Coach:

1. Clarifies the client's issues and concerns and/or opportunities for change based on the whole person assessment data.

2. Confirms the client's issues and concerns and/or opportunities with the client.

3. Tracks the client's issues and concerns and/or opportunities in a manner that leads to identification of the client's goals that will be the focus of the coaching process.

ANA Standard 3. Outcomes Identification

The registered nurse identifies expected outcomes for a plan individualized to the healthcare consumer or the situation.

Professional Nurse Coach Role

The Nurse Coach assists the client to identify goals that will lead to the desired change. The Nurse Coach values the evolution and the process of change as it unfolds.

Professional Nurse Coach Competencies

The Nurse Coach:

1. Involves the client in formulating goals that are specific, measurable, action-oriented, realistic, and time-lined.

2. Facilitates the client's process of self-discovery related to establishment of the client's goals.

3. Facilitates the client's exploration of alternative ideas and options relevant to goal-setting.

4. Supports the client's inner wisdom, intuition, and innate ability for knowing what is best for self.

5. Realizes that new goals will emerge as the client changes and evolves.

ANA Standard 4. Planning

The registered nurse develops a plan that prescribes strategies and alternatives to attain expected outcomes.

Professional Nurse Coach Role

The Nurse Coach and the client develop a coaching plan that identifies strategies to attain goals.

Professional Nurse Coach Competencies

The Nurse Coach:

1. Assists the client to identify strategies to attain goals.

2. Creates with the client an action plan with clearly defined steps and anticipated results.

3. Explores with the client potential obstacles to goal attainment and possible responses to these challenges.

4. Adjusts plan as desired by the client.

ANA Standard 5. Implementation

The registered nurse implements the identified plan.

Professional Nurse Coach Role

The Nurse Coach supports the client's coaching plan while simultaneously remaining open to emerging goals based on new insights, learning, and achievements. The Nurse Coach supports the client in reaching for new and expanded goals. The Nurse Coach utilizes a variety of specific coaching and communication skills to facilitate learning and growth.

Professional Nurse Coach Competencies

The Nurse Coach:

Before the coaching interaction:

1. Becomes fully present, centered, and grounded.

2. Reviews client status and/or progress from previously obtained data.

3. Minimizes distractions for self and encourages client to do the same.

At the beginning of the coaching interaction:

4. Explores, with the client, an outcome for the coaching session that is achievable in the time allotted.

5. Briefly explores progress since last coaching session, with particular attention to accomplishments, challenges, or barriers relevant to current session.

Throughout the coaching interaction:

6. Remains fully present, centered, and grounded.

    a. Supports the client in directing the agenda/focus of the coaching session.

    b. Acknowledges the client and identifies strengths for change.

    c. Maintains an interested, open, and reflective approach to the client.

    d. Is comfortable with silence or pausing to assist the client with reflection and finding new understanding or next steps.

    e. Accesses and trusts her/his own intuition and perceptions of the client.

    f. Draws upon the precepts of the human energy field/system to assist client in achievement of goals.

7. Creates a safe, supportive environment that fosters intimacy and trust.

8. Continuously exhibits authenticity (honesty, sincerity, personal integrity).

9. Demonstrates respect for client's subjective experiences/story, perceptions, learning style, and culture (e.g., beliefs, values, and customs).

10. Provides ongoing support for new ideas, behaviors, and actions that may involve risk-taking and fear of failure and/or fear of success.

11. Obtains the client's consent to coach client in areas of vulnerability.

12. Chooses what is most effective in the moment from a variety of coaching strategies and implements as appropriate.

13. Focuses on what the client is saying and is not saying to understand the meaning in the context of the client's desires and to support the client's self-expression by employing such skills as deep listening, relevant use of language, powerful questioning, and direct communication.

    a. Deep Listening

        i. Accepts, explores, reinforces, and encourages the client's expression of perceptions, concerns, beliefs, suggestions, etc.

        ii. Recognizes incongruities between body language, words used, and the tone of voice.

        iii. Paraphrases, reiterates, and summarizes what the client has said to ensure understanding and clarity.

        iv. Focuses on the essence of the client's communication when the client becomes involved in long explanatory descriptions.

        v. Allows the client to express strong feelings without judgment in order to facilitate movement towards achievement of goals.

        vi. Acknowledges the client's ambivalence to change and helps identify barriers.

Appendix A. The Art and Science of Nurse Coaching, 1st Edition

b. Relevant Use of Language

   i. Uses language, including metaphors and analogies, which assist the client to explore perspectives, uncertainties, or opportunities for change.

   ii. Uses language that is nonjudgmental, appropriate, and respectful.

   iii. Uses language that reflects the client's worldview, beliefs, and values.

c. Powerful Questioning

   i. Asks open-ended questions that create greater insight, clarity, and/or new possibilities and learning.

   ii. Asks questions that move the client towards desired goals.

   iii. Asks questions that evoke discovery, insight, commitment or action (e.g., those that challenge the client's assumptions).

   iv. Uses inquiry for greater awareness, clarity, and understanding.

d. Direct Communication

   i. Provides feedback in a clear and direct manner.

   ii. Shares insights with client in ways that are practical and meaningful.

   iii. Explores the client's assumptions and perspectives to evoke new ideas and discover new possibilities for action.

   iv. Challenges the client to stretch and be challenged, while maintaining a comfortable pace with the client.

14. Employs integrated, holistic communication skills including deep listening, relevant use of language, powerful questions, and direct communication, allowing the client to fully explore and articulate what she or he hopes to achieve through the coaching relationship.

  a. Supports the client's inner wisdom, intuition, and innate ability for learning.

  b. Identifies with the client additional areas for learning and development.

  c. Assists the client in uncovering underlying ambivalence, concerns, typical and fixed ways of perceiving self and the world, interpretations of experiences, and differences between thoughts, feelings, and actions.

  d. Helps the client identify barriers to change.

  e. Helps the client identify strengths and opportunities for learning and growth.

  f. Acknowledges client resistance as an opportunity for self-awareness and growth.

  g. Shares information with client that inspires broader perspectives.

  h. Encourages and supports the client to experiment and to apply what has been learned from the coaching interaction.

  i. Assists the client to determine actions that will enable the client to demonstrate, practice, and deepen new learning.

  j. Facilitates the client in taking action that will most effectively lead to achievement of desired goals and prevent relapse.

At the end of the coaching interaction:

15. Inquires of the client if the coaching session outcomes have been achieved.

16. Identifies the connection between where the client is and where she/he wishes to go.

17. Identifies with the client the next specific action steps and a timeline that will lead to achievement of desired goals.

18. Assists the client to manage progress by holding the client accountable for stated actions, results, and related time frames, while maintaining a positive and trusting relationship with the client.

19. Determines with the client when the next coaching interaction will occur.

20. Periodically, if relevant, prepares, organizes, and reviews information, including past and current actions, with the client that promotes achievement of client goals.

21. Periodically, as indicated, reviews and revises the coaching plan with the client.

22. Ends the coaching interaction in an energetic, positive, and supportive manner.

ANA Standard 6. Evaluation

The registered nurse evaluates progress toward attainment of outcomes.

Professional Nurse Coach Role

The Nurse Coach partners with the client to evaluate progress toward attainment of goals.

Professional Nurse Coach Competencies

The Nurse Coach:

1. Assists the client to evaluate effectiveness of strategies in relation to the client's responses and the attainment of the expected and unfolding goals.

2. Supports client autonomy by recognizing the client is the determinant of progress and success.

3. Documents evaluation of progress and attainment of coaching goals.

Professional Nurse Coach Performance Competencies

ANA Standard 7. Ethics

The registered nurse practices ethically.

Professional Nurse Coach Role

The Nurse Coach integrates ethical provisions in all coaching interactions.

Professional Nurse Coach Competencies

The Nurse Coach:

1. Uses *Code of Ethics for Nurses with Interpretive Statements* (ANA, 2001) to guide practice and communicate the foundation of professional Nurse Coaching practice.

2. Clearly communicates to the client and others the distinctions among coaching, consulting, counseling, and teaching.

3. Provides coaching in a manner that recognizes and respects the client's autonomy, dignity, rights, values, and beliefs.

4. Maintains an effective coaching relationship that is congruent with the coaching agreement and within the boundaries of professional nursing practice.

5. Values all life experiences as opportunities to find personal meaning and cultivate self-awareness, self-reflection, and growth.

6. Maintains client confidentiality within legal and regulatory parameters.

ANA Standard 8. Education

The registered nurse attains knowledge and competence that reflects current nursing practice.

Professional Nurse Coach Role

The Nurse Coach attains knowledge and competence that reflects current Nurse Coaching practice.

Professional Nurse Coach Competencies

The Nurse Coach:

1. Participates in ongoing educational activities to enhance the Nurse Coaching role.

2. Documents and maintains evidence of Nurse Coaching competence.

3. Develops and uses a broad knowledge base related to holistic/integral nursing, integrative health, health systems, professional coaching competencies, counseling, health education, health promotion, and nursing practice issues.

ANA Standard 9. Evidence-Based Practice and Research

The registered nurse integrates evidence and research findings into practice.

Professional Nurse Coach Role

The Nurse Coach integrates evidence and research into Nurse Coaching practice.

Professional Nurse Coach Competencies

The Nurse Coach:

1. Uses the best available evidence, including theories and research findings, to guide and enhance professional Nurse Coaching practice.

2. Participates with others to establish research priorities and to identify research questions or areas for inquiry related to professional Nurse Coaching practice.

3. Participates in research activities related to professional Nurse Coaching practice.

ANA Standard 10. Quality of Practice
The registered nurse contributes to quality nursing practice.

Professional Nurse Coach Role
The Nurse Coach systematically enhances the quality and effectiveness of Nurse Coaching practice.

Professional Nurse Coach Competencies
The Nurse Coach:
Participates in quality improvement to enhance Nurse Coaching practice.

1. Contributes to the education of others concerning Nurse Coaching practice.

2. Documents Nurse Coaching interactions in a responsible, accountable, and ethical manner to facilitate quality review and promotion of effective Nurse Coaching practice.

3. Uses creativity and innovation in Nurse Coaching practice to improve client outcomes.

4. Analyzes organizational systems for barriers to effective implementation of Nurse Coaching practice.

5. Advocates use of *The Art and Science of Nurse Coaching: The Provider's Guide to Coaching Scope and Competencies* to evaluate and enhance the quality of practice.

ANA Standard 11. Communication

The registered nurse communicates effectively in a variety of formats in all areas of practice.

Professional Nurse Coach Role

The Nurse Coach employs skillful communication in all aspects of the coaching interaction.

Professional Nurse Coach Competencies

The Nurse Coach:

1. Understands that skillful communication is a fundamental component of professional Nurse Coaching practice.

2. Communicates, when requested by client, with family, significant others, caregivers, healthcare providers, and others to assist and enhance the client's achievement of coaching goals.

ANA Standard 12. Leadership

The registered nurse demonstrates leadership in the professional practice setting and the profession.

Professional Nurse Coach Role

The Nurse Coach demonstrates leadership in the promotion of effective Nurse Coaching for clients.

Professional Nurse Coach Competencies

The Nurse Coach:

1. Advances the role of the Nurse Coach among health professional and coaching colleagues and in professional organizations.

2. Develops cognitive, emotional, moral, and spiritual intelligence to enhance leadership skills.

3. Promotes the success of others by using effective Nurse Coaching interventions.

4. Demonstrates energy, excitement, and a passion for quality Nurse Coaching.

5. Willingly accepts that mistakes will be made by self and others when taking risks to achieve goals.

6. Displays the ability to define a clear vision, associated goals, and a plan to implement and measure progress toward goals.

Appendix A. *The Art and Science of Nurse Coaching, 1st Edition*

ANA Standard 13. Collaboration

The registered nurse collaborates with healthcare consumer, family, and others in the conduct of nursing practice.

Professional Nurse Coach Role

The Nurse Coach collaborates with others to assist clients in achieving goals.

Professional Nurse Coach Competencies

The Nurse Coach:

1. Uses effective communication and change skills with individuals and groups to collaboratively identify and achieve individual, group, and organizational goals.

2. Works collaboratively with other health and wellness coaches in interprofessional development initiatives.

3. Collaborates with others to promote Nurse Coaching as a way to enhance client outcomes.

ANA Standard 14. Professional Practice Evaluation

The registered nurse evaluates her or his own nursing practice in relation to professional practice standards and guidelines, relevant statutes, and regulations.

Professional Nurse Coach Role

The Nurse Coach evaluates her or his own Nurse Coaching practice in relation to professional practice standards and guidelines, relevant statutes, rules, and regulations. The Nurse Coach is engaged in ongoing personal and professional self-development.

Professional Nurse Coach Competencies

The Nurse Coach:

1. Utilizes *The Art and Science of Nurse Coaching: The Provider's Guide to Coaching Scope and Competencies* to evaluate and enhance quality of practice.

2. Considers the effect of one's personal values, culture, spiritual beliefs, experiences, biases, and education on the provision of Nurse Coaching services to individuals, groups, and organizations.

3. Provides Nurse Coaching services in a manner that is appropriate and sensitive to culture and ethnicity.

4. Engages in self-evaluation of Nurse Coaching practice on a regular basis, identifying areas of strength as well as areas in which additional development would be beneficial.

5. Obtains evaluative feedback regarding one's own coaching from clients, peers, and professional colleagues and takes appropriate action based upon the feedback.

6. Pursues professional Nurse Coach certification as a way to demonstrate competence and to promote the Nurse Coaching role to employers, clients, and the public.

7. Recognizes that Nurse Coaching practice is enhanced by ongoing self-development to promote physical, mental, emotional, social, moral, and spiritual well-being.

8. Receives personal and professional coaching to enhance quality of Nurse Coaching practice.

9. Integrates knowledge from research on coaching into practice.

ANA Standard 15. Resource Utilization

The registered nurse utilizes appropriate resources to plan and provide nursing services that are safe, effective, and financially responsible.

Professional Nurse Coach Role

The Nurse Coach considers factors related to safety, effectiveness, cost, and impact on practice in the planning and delivery of Nurse Coaching services.

Professional Nurse Coach Competencies

The Nurse Coach:

1. Evaluates factors such as safety, effectiveness, availability, cost and benefits, efficiencies, and impact on Nurse Coaching practice when suggesting options for the client that would result in the same expected outcome.

2. Assists the client, as appropriate, in identifying and securing appropriate and available services to facilitate achievement of client goals.

ANA Standard 16. Environmental Health
The registered nurse practices in an environmentally safe and healthy manner.

Professional Nurse Coach Role
The Nurse Coach considers the impact of the internal and external environment of self and client when providing Nurse Coaching services.

Professional Nurse Coach Competencies
The Nurse Coach:

1. Understands that healthy environments encompass both internal and external environments

2. Recognizes that individual (physical, psychological, emotional, spiritual) and cultural, social, and historical factors influence internal and external environments.

3 Considers the internal and external healing environments of self and client regarding contribution to client goal achievement.

Glossary

Source: Used with permission and adapted from Dossey & Keegan, 2013.

Active imagination. A process of conscious formation of images by the client as a technique or method to access deeper information and personal wisdom to facilitate changes; may include guided imagery.

Bearing witness. Being present for things as they are with the client or another; a state and skills that are achieved and learned through reflective practice (relaxation, prayer, meditation, nature walks) that can shift an experience of separateness to one of connection; it involves developing the qualities of stillness in order to be present for others.

Deep listening. The communication between two or more individuals in which the conventional division of self and ego is transcended by a sense of indivisible unity between all involved. Deep listening involves being present, allowing space and being focused with intention to understand what another person is expressing or not expressing (Dossey, Luck, & Schaub, 2013).

Emotional intelligence. The ability to perceive emotion in self and others; the ability to use emotions as a source of information; the ability to comprehend the complex relationships among emotions; and the ability to manage emotions to achieve desired outcomes. Emotional intelligence is concerned with understanding self and others and being able to relate to others. Emotional intelligence requires attunement to social norms. Emotional intelligence is a learned capability.

Environment. The context of habitat within which all living systems participate and interact, including the physical body and its physical habitat along with the cultural, psychological, social, and historical influences; includes both the external physical space and the person's internal physical, mental, emotional, social, and spiritual experience.

Environmental determinants of health. Any external agent (biological, chemical, physical, social, or cultural) that can be linked to a change in health status that is involuntary, i.e. breathing unwanted secondhand smoke, whereas active tobacco smoking is a behavioral determinant.

Ethics. The basic underlying concept of the unity and integral wholeness of all people and all of nature, identified and pursued by finding unity and wholeness within the self and within humanity. In this framework, acts are not performed for the sake of law, precedent, or social norms, but rather from a desire to do good freely in order to witness, identify, and contribute to unity.

Evidence-based practice. The process by which healthcare practitioners make clinical decisions using the best philosophy and theories, research evidence, clinical expertise, and patient preferences within the context of available resources.

Healing. The lifelong journey seeking harmony and balance in one's own life and in one's family, community, and global relations. Healing involves those physical, mental, social, and spiritual processes of recovery, repair, renewal, and transformation that increase wholeness and often (though not invariably) order and coherence. Healing is an emergent process of the whole system bringing together aspects of one's self and the body-mind-emotion-spirit-environment at deeper levels of inner knowing, leading toward integration and balance, with each aspect having equal importance and value. Healing can lead to more complex levels of personal understanding and meaning, and may be synchronous but not synonymous with curing. It is a sense of contentment with what is and a freedom from struggle.

Healing intention. The conscious awareness of being in the present moment to help facilitate the healing process; a volitional act of unconditional love.

Healing process. A continual journey of changing and evolving of one's self through life that is characterized by the awareness of patterns that support or are challenges/barriers to health and healing. This journey may be done alone or in a healing community. The healing process may occur until a person's final breath.

Healing relationships. The quality and characteristics of interactions between two people towards harmony and balance such as empathy, caring, love, warmth, trust, confidence, credibility, competence, honesty, courtesy, respect, sharing expectations, and a heart-to-heart connection.

Health. An individually defined state or process in which the individual (nurse, person, family, group, or community) experiences a sense of growth, well-being, harmony, and unity such that subjective experiences about health, health beliefs, and values are honored; a process of becoming an expanding consciousness.

Health promotion. Activities and preventive measures to facilitate growth, promote health, increase well-being, and actualize human potential of people, families, communities, society, and ecology such as immunizations, fitness/exercise programs, breast self-exams, appropriate nutrition, relaxation, stress management, social support, prayer, meditation, healing rituals, cultural practices, and promotion of environmental health and safety.

Holistic. Based on an understanding that patient is an interconnected unity and that physical, mental, emotional, social, spiritual, and environmental factors need to be included in any interventions. The whole is a system that is greater than the sum of its parts.

Holistic communication. A free flow of verbal and nonverbal interchange between and among people and significant beings such as pets, nature, and God/Life Force/Absolute/Transcendent that explores meaning and ideas leading to mutual understanding and growth.

Human caring. The moral ideal of nursing in which the nurse brings one's entire self into a relationship with the whole self of the client in order to protect the client's vulnerability, preserve her or his humanity and dignity, and reinforce the meaning and experience of oneness and unity.

Integral. A comprehensive synthesizing framework or multidimensional perspective. An integral approach addresses all levels of human experience (subjective and objective; individual and collective) in a combined, synergistic manner.

Integrative. An approach that puts the client at the center and addresses the whole person and full range of physical, emotional, mental, social, spiritual and environmental influences that affect health; includes the client's personalized action plan to maintain optimal health behaviors and human flourishing, and to heal illness and disease.

Intuition. The perceived knowing of things and events without the conscious use of rational processes; using all the senses to receive and process information.

Moral intelligence. The mental capacity to apply universal human principles, such as integrity, responsibility, compassion and forgiveness, to personal values, goals, and actions.

Not-knowing. Being free of fixed ideas.

Nurse Coach. A registered nurse who integrates coaching competencies into any setting or specialty area of practice to facilitate a process of change or development that assists individuals or groups to realize their potential.

Nurse Coaching. A skilled, purposeful, results-oriented, and structured relationship-centered interaction with clients provided by registered nurses for the purpose of promoting achievement of client goals.

Nurse Coaching process. An iterative process that involves six steps that may occur simultaneously. (1) Establish relationship and assess client readiness for change; (2) Identify opportunities and issues; (3) Assist client to establish goals; (4) Structure the coaching interaction; (5) Empower clients to reach goals, and; (6) Assist client to determine extent to which goals were achieved.

Presence. The condition of being consciously and compassionately in the present moment with another, believing in her or his inherent wholeness, whatever the current situation; the essence of nursing care; the gift of self. Presence involves: approaching an individual or a situation in a way that respects and honors; relating in a way that reflects a quality of being with and in collaboration with; entering into a shared experience (or field of consciousness) that promotes growth, healing, and an experience of well-being. Presence is a combination of attributes that include intentionality, mutuality, client centeredness, and attending. Presence is a nursing intervention. Presence transforms experiences, adds a deeper, more powerful dimension, reduces anxiety and promotes a nurturing atmosphere. Presence is trying to understand the meaning of an experience for another without judgment. Presence is a way of being that involves connection so that growth and healing are promoted for self and others. Presence is necessary for genuine and empathetic communication.

Social determinants of health. The economic and social conditions under which individuals live that affect their health; disease and illness are often a result of detrimental social, economic, and political forces.

Spiritual intelligence. The recognition that physical reality is embedded within a larger, multidimensional reality with which we interact, knowingly or unknowingly. This larger reality includes and transcends the ego and the physical body. Spiritual intelligence involves the ability to act with compassion and wisdom, while maintaining inner and outer peace, regardless of circumstances. Spiritual intelligence includes the ability to access one's deepest meanings and highest motivations. It is the intelligence we use to determine that one course of action is more meaningful than another.

Suffering. An individual's experience of struggle based on a reinforced story around anxiety, distress, or pain. It can manifest as behavioral, emotional, mental, moral, physical, social and/or spiritual signs of distress; it is anguish experienced—internally and externally—as a threat to one's composure, integrity, sense of self, or the fulfillment of expectations.

Transpersonal. A personal understanding that is based on one's experiences of temporarily transcending or moving beyond one's usual identification with the limited biological, historical, cultural, and personal self at the deepest and most profound levels of experience possible. From this perspective the ordinary, biological, historical, cultural,. and personal self is seen as an important but only a partial manifestation or expression of this much greater something that is one's deeper origin and destination. It is that which transcends the limits and boundaries of individual ego identities and possibilities to include acknowledgment and appreciation of something greater (Schaub & Schaub, 2013).

Wellness. A desirable quality of life that provides satisfaction; a multidimensional state of existence experienced as well-being; integrated, congruent functioning aimed toward reaching one's highest potential.

Vulnerability. A universal human awareness that our physical lives are transitory; an awareness that can serve as a bridge among all peoples (Schaub & Schaub, 1997).

References

American Association of Colleges of Nursing (AACN). (2011). *Fact sheet.* Retrieved from: http://www.aacn.nche.edu/Media/FactSheets/nursfact. htm

American Holistic Nurses Association and American Nurses Association (AHNA/ANA). (2013). *Holistic nursing: Scope and standards of practice.* (2nd ed.) Silver Spring, MD: Nursesbooks.org.

American Holistic Nurses Credentialing Corporation (AHNCC). AHNCC Nurse Coach Certification. Retrieved from http://www.ahncc.org/ certification/nursecoachnchwnc.html

American Nurses Association (ANA) (2001.) *Code of Ethics for Nurses with interpretive statements.* Washington, DC: Nursesbooks.org.

American Nurses Association (ANA). (2010a). *Nursing: Scope and standards of nursing practice* (2nd ed.) Silver Spring, MD: Nursesbooks.org.

American Nurses Association (ANA). (2010b). *Nursing's social policy statement: The essence of the profession.* Silver Spring, MD: Nursesbooks. org.

Antonovsky, A. (1996). The salutogenic model as a theory to guide health promotion. *Health Promotion International, 11*(1), 11–18.

Atkinson, P. A., Martin, C. R., & Rankin, J. (2009). Resilience revisited. *Journal of Psychiatric and Mental Health Nursing, 16,* 137–145.

Baldwin, C. M., Schultz, A. A., Melnyk, B. M., & Rycroft-Malone, J. (2013). Evidence-based nursing practice. In B.M. Dossey & L. Keegan, *Holistic Nursing: A Handbook for Practice* (6th ed.), (pp. 797–814). Burlington, MA: Jones & Bartlett Learning.

Bandura, A. (1977). Self-efficacy: Toward a unifying theory of behavioral change. *Psychological Review* 84(2), 191, 215.

Bark Coaching Institute. (n.d.). *A path to learning successful coaching.* Retrieved from http://www.barkcoaching.com/coaching.html

Bark L. (2011). *The wisdom of the whole: Coaching for joy, health, and success.* San Francisco, CA: Create Space.

Barrett, E. A. M. (1983). *An empirical investigation of Martha E. Rogers' principle of helicy: The relationship of human field motion and power.* Unpublished doctoral dissertation, New York University, New York.

Barrett, E. A. M. (1989). A nursing theory of power for nursing practice: Derivation from Rogers' paradigm. In J. Riehl (Ed.). *Conceptual models for nursing practice* (3rd ed.). (pp. 207–217). Norwalk, CT: Appleton & Lange.

Barrett, E.A.M. (2003). Update on a measure of power as knowing participation in change. In O. L. Strickland & C. DiIorio (Eds.), Vol. 4. *Measurement of nursing outcomes: Focus on patient/client outcomes* (pp. 21–39). New York: Springer.

Becker, M. (1990). Theoretical models of adherence and strategies for improving adherence. In S. A. Shumaker, E.B. Schron, & J. K. Ockene (Eds.), *The handbook of human health behavior* (pp. 5–43). New York: Springer.

Benner, P. (1985). The oncology clinical specialist: An expert coach. *Oncology Nursing Forum 12*, 40–4.

Benner, P. (1984), *Novice to expert: Excellence and power in clinical nursing practice.* Menlo Park, CA: Addison-Wesley.

Carper, B. A, (1978). Fundamental patterns of knowing in nursing. *Advances in Nursing Science 1*(1), 13–23.

CGFNS International. Retrieved from http://www.cgfns.org/sections/about/

Chenoweth, L., Gallagher, R. Sheriff, J. N., Donoghue, J., & Stein-Parbury, J. (2008). Factors supporting self-management in Parkinson's disease: Implications for nursing practice. *International Journal of Older People Nursing, 3*, 187-193.

Cooperrider, D. L. & Whitney, D. (2005). *Appreciative inquiry: A positive revolution in change.* San Francisco, CA: Berrett-Koehler.

Cooperrider, D. L., Whitney, D., & Stavros, J. M. (2005). *Appreciative inquiry handbook.* Brunswick, OH: Crown Custom.

Cowling, R. (2001). Unitary appreciative inquiry. *Advanced Nursing Science, 23*(4), 32-48.

Csikszentmihalyi, M. (1990). *Flow: The psychology of optimal experience.* New York: Harper and Row.

Dart, M.A. (2011). *Motivational interviewing in nursing practice.* Sudbury, MA: Jones and Bartlett Learning.

Donner, G., & Wheeler, M. (2009). *Coaching in nursing: An introduction.* Indianapolis, IN: International Council of Nursing & Sigma Theta Tau. Retrieved from. http.//www.nursingsociety.org/Education/ProfessionalDevelopment/Documents/Coaching%20and%20Mentoring%20Workbook_STTI.pdf

Dossey, B. M. (2013). Nursing: Integral, integrative, and holistic—local to global. In B.M. Dossey & L. Keegan, *Holistic Nursing: A Handbook for Practice* (6th ed.), (pp.1-57). Burlington, MA: Jones & Bartlett Learning.

Dossey, B. M. (2009). Integral and holistic nursing: Local to global. In B.M. Dossey & L. Keegan, *Holistic Nursing: A Handbook for Practice* (5th ed.), (pp. 3-46). Sudbury, MA: Jones and Bartlett Learning.

Dossey, B. M. (2010). *Florence Nightingale: Mystic, visionary, healer.* Commemorative Edition. Philadelphia: F. A. Davis.

Dossey, B. M., & Hess, D. (in press). *Professional Nurse Coach core curriculum.* (Unpublished manuscript). Available from author.

Dossey, B. M., & Keegan, L. (2013). *Holistic nursing: A handbook for practice* (6th ed.). Burlington, MA: Jones and Bartlett Learning.

Dossey, B. M., Luck, S., & Schaub, B. G. (2013). *Nurse coaching in health and wellness*. Huntington, NY: Florence Press.

Dossey, B. M., Selanders, L. C., Beck , D. M., & Attewell, A. (2005). *Florence Nightingale today: Healing, leadership, global action*. Silver Spring, MD: Nursebooks.org.

Erickson, H. L. (Ed.). (2010). *Exploring the interface between the philosophy and discipline of holistic nursing: Modeling and Role-Modeling at work*. Cedar Park, TX: Unicorns Unlimited.

Erickson, E., Tomlin, E., & Swain, M. A. (1983/2009). *Modeling and role-modeling: A theory and paradigm for nursing*. Englewood Cliffs, NJ: Prentice-Hall.

Fawcett, J. (1995). *Analysis and evaluation of conceptual models of nursing* (3rded.). Philadelphia: F. A. Davis.

Freshwater, D., Taylor, B. J., & Sherwood, G.C. (Eds.). (2008). *The international textbook of reflective practice in nursing*. Chichester, United Kingdom: Wiley-Blackwell.

Gillespie, B. M., Chaboyer, W., & Wallis, M. (2007). Development of a theoretically derived model of resilience through concept analysis. *Contemporary Nurse, 25*(1–2), 124–135.

Hatweg, D. L. & Fleck, L. M. Dorothea Orem's self-care deficit theory. In Parker, M. E. & Smith, M. C. *Nursing theories and nursing practice* (3rd ed.) (121–145). Philadelphia: F. A. Davis.

Hayes, E., & Kalmakis, K. A. (2007). From the sidelines: Coaching as a nurse practitioner strategy for improving health outcomes. *Journal of the American Academy of Nurse Practitioners, 19*(11), 555–562.

Hess, D., Bark, L., & Southard, M. E. (2010, September). White paper: Holistic Nurse Coaching. *Summit on standards & credentialing of professional coaches in healthcare & wellness*. Paper presented to National Credentialing Team for Professional Coaches in Healthcare, Boston, MA. Retrieved from http://www.ahncc.org/holisticnursecoaching.html

Hess, D. & Dossey, B. M. (In press). *Nurse coaching: A review of the literature.* (Submitted as a white paper to American Holistic Nurses Credentialing Corporation on December 16, 2011.) Available from authors.)

Hyman, M., Ornish, D., & Roizen, M. (2009). Life style medicine: Treating the causes of disease. *Alternative Therapies, 15*(6), 12–14.

Institute of Medicine. (2010). *The future of nursing: Leading change, advancing health.* Washington, DC: National Academies Press. Retrieved from http://www.iom.edu/Reports/2010/The-Future-of-Nursing-Leading-Change-Advancing-Health.aspx

Integrative Nurse Coach Certificate Program. (n.d.). *Why integrative nurse coaching?* Retrieved from http://inursecoach.com/education/why-inccp/

International Coaching Federation. (2011a), ICF core competencies. Retrieved from http://www.coachfederation.org/icfcredentials/core-competencies

International Coach Federation. (2011b). ICF stats. Retrieved from http://www.coachfederation.org/about-icf/press-room/

International Coaching Federation. (2011c). ICF Code of Ethics. Retrieved from http://www.coachfederation.org/icfcredentials/ethics/

International Council of Nurses. (n.d.)Retrieved from http://www.icn.ch/

Interprofessional Education Collaborative Expert Panel. (2011). *Core competencies for interprofessional collaborative practice: Report of an expert panel.* Washington, D.C.: Interprofessional Education Collaborative.

Johns, C. (2010). Reflection as a way-of-being in practice. In H. L. Erickson (Ed.), *Modeling and role-modeling at work,* (pp. 311–328). Cedar Park, TX: Unicorns Unlimited.

Kegan, R. & Lahey, L. L. (2009). *Immunity to change: How to overcome it and unlock the potential in yourself and your organization.* Boston: Harvard Business School Publishing.

Kimball, B., Joynt, J., Cherner, D., & O'Neil, E. (2007). The quest for new innovative care delivery models. *Journal of Nursing Administration 37*(9), 392–398.

Koerner, J. (2011). *Healing: The essence of nursing.* New York: Springer.

Kreitzer, M. J., Sierpina, V. S., & Lawson, K. (2008). Health coaching: Innovative education and clinical programs emerging. *Explore, 4*(2), 154–155.

Langeland, E., Wahl, A. K., Kristoffersen, K., & Hanestad, B. R. (2007). Promoting coping: Salutogenesis among people with mental health problems. *Issues in Mental Health Nursing, 28,* 275–295. doi: 10.1080/01612840601172627

Lawson, K. (2009). Could health coaching build a bridge to a new system of healthcare? *Alternative Therapies in Health and Medicine, 15*(5), 16–18.

Luck, S. (2010). Changing the health of our nation: The role of nurse coaches. *Alternative Therapies in Health and Medicine, 16*(5), 78–80.

McCraty R & Childres D. (2010). Coherence: Bridging personal, social, and global health. *Alternative Therapies in Health and Medicine,* 16(4), 10–24.

Mallock, K., & Porter-O'Grady, T. (2005). *The quantum leader: Applications for the new world of work.* Sudbury, MA: Jones and Bartlett.

McNally, K., & Cunningham, L. (2010). *Nurse executive's coaching manual.* Indianapolis, IN: Sigma Theta Tau International.

Meyers, D., Peikes, D., Genevro, J., Peterson, G., Taylor, E. F., Lake, T., & Grumbach, K. (2010). The roles of patient-centered medical homes and accountable care organizations in coordinating patient care. AHRQ Publication No. 11-M005-EF. Rockville, MD: Agency for Health Care Research and Quality. Retrieved from http://www.ahrq.gov/

Miller, W. R., Rollnick, S. (2002). *Motivational interviewing: Preparing people for change* (2nd ed.). New York: Guilford Press.

Moore, M. & Tschannen-Moran B. (2010). *Coaching psychology manual.* Philadelphia: Lippincott, Williams & Wilkins.

Moore, S. M., & Charvat, J. (2007). Promoting health behavior change using appreciative inquiry: Moving from deficit models to affirmation models of care. *Family and Community Health/Supplement 1, 30*(15), 564–574.

Munhall, P. L. (1993). Unknowing: Toward another pattern of knowing in nursing. *Nursing Outlook 41* (3), 125–128.

National Consortium for the Credentialing of Health and Wellness Coaches. (NCCHWC). 2010. National Summit on Standards and Credentialing of Professional Coaches in Healthcare and Wellness. September 26-27, 2010. Retrieved from http://www.ncchwc.org/files/SummitSundayPPT.pdf

National Consortium for the Credentialing of Health and Wellness Coaches (NCCHWC). (2011) *Progress report.* July. Retrieved from http://www.wellcoaches.com/images/pdf/progressreport-nationalteam-jul-2011.pdf

National Prevention Council (2011). *National Prevention Strategy: American's plan for better health and wellness.* Washington, DC: U.S. Department of Health and Human Services, Office of the Surgeon General. Retrieved from http://www.cdc.gov/policy/nps/

National Prevention Council (2012). *National Prevention Council Action Plan* Washington, DC: U.S. Department of Health and Human Services, Office of the Surgeon General. (2012). Retrieved from http://www.cdc.gov/policy/nps/

Newman, M. A. (1986). *Health as expanding consciousness.* St. Louis, MO: C.V. Mosby.

Newman, M. A. (1994). *Health as expanding consciousness.* (2nd ed.). St. Louis, MO: C.V. Mosby.

Neuman, B., & Fawcett, J. (Eds.). (2010). *The Neuman Systems Model* (5th ed.). Upper Saddle River, NJ: Pearson.

Nightingale, F. (1859). *Notes on hospitals.* London, England: John W. Parker.

Nightingale, F. (1860). *Notes on nursing: What it is and what it is not.* London, England: Harrison.

Nightingale, F. (1893). Sick-nursing and health-nursing. In B. Coutts (Ed.), *Woman's Mission* (pp. 184–205). London, England: Sampson, Low, Marston.

Nightingale Declaration for a Healthy World. Retrieved from http://www.nightingaledeclaration.net/the-declaration

Nursing Interventions Classification (NIC) (n.d.). NIC labels and definitions. Retrieved from http://www.nursing.uiowa.edu/cncce/nic-labels-and-definitions [Source: Bulechek, G.M., Butcher, H. K., & Dochterman, J.C. (Eds.). (2008). *Nursing Interventions Classification (NIC)* (5th ed.). St. Louis, MO: Mosby Elsevier.]

Orem, D. E. (1971). *Nursing concepts of practice*. New York: McGraw Hill.

Patient Protection and Affordable Care Act, H. R. 3590. Pub. L. No. 111–148 (2010). Retrieved from http://democrats.senate.gov/pdfs/reform/patient-protection-affordable-care-act-as-passed.pdf

Parse, R. R. (1981). *Man-living-health: A theory of nursing*. New York: John Wiley and Sons.

Parse, R. R. (1995). *Illuminations: The human becoming theory in practice and research*. New York: National League for Nursing Press.

Peplau, H. E. (1952). *Interpersonal relations in nursing*. New York: G. P. Putnam's Sons.

Potter, P., & Frisch, N. C, (2013). The nursing process. In Dossey, B. M. & Keegan, L. *Holistic nursing: A handbook for practice* (6th ed.) (145–160). Burlington, MA: Jones and Bartlett Learning

Prochaska, J.O., Norcross, J.C., & DeClemente, C.C. (1995). *Changing for good: A revolutionary six-stage program for overcoming bad habits and moving your life positively forward*. New York: Harper Collins.

Rogers, M. E. (1970). *An introduction to the theoretical basis of nursing*. Philadelphia, PA: F. A. Davis.

Rollnick, S., Miller, W.R., & Butler, C. C. (2008). *Motivational interviewing in healthcare: Helping patients change behavior*. New York: Guilford Press.

Roy, C. (2009). *The Roy Adaptation Model* (3rd ed.) Upper Saddle River, NJ: Prentice-Hall Health.

Samueli Institute. (2008). *Wellness initiative for the nation*. Alexandria, VA: Author. Retrieved from http://www.samueliinstitute.org/health-policy/wellness-initiative-for-the-nation-win

Schaub, B. G., Luck, S., & Dossey, B. M. (2012). Integrative nurse coaching for health and wellness. *Alternative and Complementary Therapies, 18*(1), 14–20.

Schaub, B.G. & Schaub, R. (1997). *Healing addictions: The vulnerability model of recovery.* Albany, NY: Delmar Publishers.

Schaub, R., & Schaub, B.G. (2009). *The end of fear: A spiritual path for realists.* Carlsbad, CA: Hay House.

Schaub, R. & Schaub, B. G. (2013). *Transpersonal development: Cultivating the human resources of peace, wisdom, purpose and oneness.* Huntington, NY: Florence Press.

Scholle, S.H., Torda, P., Peikes, D., Han, E., & Genevro, J. (2010). *Engaging patients and families in the medical home.* AHRQ Publication No. 10-0083-EF. Rockville, MD: Agency for Health Care Research and Quality. Retrieved from http://www.ahrq.gov/

Schenck, S. (2002). Nurse coach: Healthcare resource for this millennium. *Nursing Forum, 37*(3), 14–20.

Seligman, M. E. P. (1990). Learned optimism: How to change your mind and your life. New York: Free Press.

Sigma Theta Tau International. (n.d.)Retrieved from http://www.nursingsociety.org/aboutus/mission/Pages/factsheet.aspx

Southard, M. E. (2003). *A new provider for the new healthcare industry: The Nurse Coach.* (Unpublished manuscript). Available from author.

Snyderman, R., & Dinan, M. (2010). Improving health by taking it personally. *Journal of the American Medical Association, 303*(4), 363–364.

United Nations. (2011). Millennium Development Goals Report 2011. Retrieved from http://www.un.org/millenniumgoals/

U.S. Department of Health and Human Services, Office of Disease Prevention and Health Promotion, (n.d.). Introducing Healthy People 2020. Retrieved from http://www.healthypeople.gov/2020/about/default.aspx

Warelow, E. K. (2005). Resilience: When coping is emotionally intelligent. *Journal of the American Psychiatric Nurses Association, 11*(2), 101–2.

Watson Caring Science Institute. (n.d.). *Caritas coaching education program.* Retrieved from http://www.watsoncaringscience.org/index.cfm/ category/3/caritas-coach-education-program-ccep.cfm

Watson, J. (1985). *Nursing: Human science and human caring: A theory of nursing.* Norwalk, CT: Appleton and Lange.

Watson, J. (2007). *Nursing human science and human care: A theory of nursing.* Sudbury, MA: Jones and Bartlett Learning.

White, J. (1995). Patterns of knowing: Review, critique, and update. *Advances in Nursing Science* 17(2), 73–86.

Wilson, M. (2009). Complexity theory. *Whitireia Nursing Journal,* (16), 18–24.

Wolever, R. Q., & Eisenberg, D. M. (2011). What is health coaching anyway? Standards needed to enable rigorous research. *Archives of Internal Medicine.* doi:10.1001/archinternmed.2011.508. Retrieved from http:// archinte.jamanetwork.com/article.aspx?articleid=1106048

World Health Organization. (2009). *World Health Organization statistics report 2009.* Retrieved from http://www.learningnurse.com/content/ view/34/49/

World Health Organization. (2011). United Nations high-level meeting on noncommunicable disease prevention and control, September 2011. Retrieved from www.who.int/nmh/publications/ncd_profiles2011/en/ index.html

World Health Organization. (n.d.) Global Network of WHO Collaborating Centres (WHOCCs). Retrieved from http://www.parlatore.com.br/whocc/

Zahourek, R. P. (2013). Holistic nursing research: Challenges and opportunities. In B. M. Dossey & L. Keegan, *Holistic nursing: A handbook for practice* (6th ed.), (pp. 775–796). Burlington, MA: Jones & Bartlett Learning.

Appendix A.

Background

Formation of the Professional Nurse Coaching Workgroup (PNCW)

The Art and Science of Nurse Coaching: The Provider's Guide to Coaching Scope and Competencies is the product of significant exploratory conversations and electronic mail communication among the Professional Nurse Coach Workgroup (PNCW) (see the Contributors section for the members of this workgroup) over a three-year period and involving a six-step process.

Clarifying the Role of the Nurse Coach

During the initial PNCW meetings, foundational concepts of Nurse Coaching and the Nurse Coach role as a component of nursing practice were discussed. These discussions also included the growing emergence of nonprofessional health and wellness coaches as well as the development of health and wellness coaches in other professions. In September 2010, the PNCW circulated *White Paper on Holistic Nurse Coaching* (Hess, Bark, & Southard, 2010). All PNCW members attended the National Summit on Standards and Credentialing of Professional Coaches in Healthcare and Wellness (NCCHWC) convened by the National Consortium for the Credentialing of Health and Wellness Coaches Progress Report in Boston, Massachusetts, in Boston, Massachusetts, to explore the future of health and wellness coaches (NCCHWC, 2010; 2011). *The Art and Science of Nurse Coaching* has been developed by nurse coaching experts and vetted via a thorough peer-review process to fully describe the professional Nurse Coach role.

Initiating Nursing Alliances

The PNCW entered into a conversation regarding the importance of the role of the Nurse Coach and the need for a national certification process for Nurse Coaches with the American Holistic Nurse Credentialing Corporation (AHNCC). After lengthy discussion, the PNCW entered an agreement with

AHNCC whereby AHNCC would sponsor the work of the PNCW in exchange for the rights to establish a national certification process for the Nurse Coach. The Nurse Coach Certification process is voluntary. Nurses integrate Nurse Coach competencies in accordance with *Nursing: Scope and Standards of Practice*, 2nd Edition (ANA, 2010a). (See Appendix B.)

The PNCW and many nurse leaders continued to be engaged in conversations related to alliances with other interprofessional organizations (Interprofessional Education Collaborative Expert Panel, 2011; NCCHWEC, 2011) (see Steps 4 and 5 below) for the purpose of establishing clear guidelines and competencies for professional health and wellness coaches.

Articulating the Nurse Coach's Scope of Practice and Competencies and Six-Step Process

The creation of *The Art and Science of Nurse Coaching* is the successful completion of a three-year process. The PNCW engaged with a Review Committee and an Advisory Committee. (For the individuals who served on these and other groups involved in the process, see the Contributors section on pages vii and viii.) The following describes the extensive six-step course of action.

Step 1: Literature Review

The six-member PNCW conducted an extensive literature review regarding Nurse Coaching from 2009–2011. The goals were to: (1) Identify how the health and wellness coach role was embedded in nursing practice; (2) Identify areas where Nurse Coaching skills were used and integrated; (3) Determine how Nurse Coaches defined their roles, practices, and competencies; (4) Explore emerging trends within professional Nurse Coaching practice; and (5) Identify areas of future research in Nurse Coaching.

Step 2: The Compilation Process

Following Step 1 and during 2010–2011, the six-member PNCW compiled and reviewed the literature and discussed findings. Following a series of meetings, they drafted *Professional Nurse Coach Role: Defining Scope of Practice and Competencies*. The current retitled document is the result of extensive reviews and several revisions by the PNCW members.

Concurrently, and in preparation for Steps 3 and 4, the PNCW compiled a list of expert nurses engaged in coaching for the Review Committee and for the Advisory Committee.

Step 3: Review Committee

The expert Review Committee was provided with *The Art and Science of Nurse Coaching* and was directed to review and strengthen the document by providing additional comments, deletions, modifications, and recommendations. The revised draft document was again sent to the Review Committee for additional comments, deletions, modifications, and recommendations.

Step 4: Advisory Committee

The Advisory Committee was also provided with *The Art and Science of Nurse Coaching* and followed the same process as the Review Committee. The PNCW directive to the Advisory Committee also included the identification of strategies to obtain national and global nursing organizations endorsement (Step 5).

Step 5: Steps Toward Official ANA Document and Endorsing Organizations

The revised draft of *The Art and Science of Nurse Coaching* was sent to ANA on December 1, 2011 to begin the steps towards an officially recognized ANA document. As soon as this process was completed (in early 2012) the document was sent to their 28 affiliate organizations. The PNCW has followed the recommendations of ANA and the Advisory Board regarding contact with other national and global nursing organizations. The CGFNS International was the first global endorsing organization. As organizations responded with endorsement they were added to the list that appears in the Contributors section on page ix.

Step 6: Development of Core Curriculum for Professional Nurse Coaching Practice

Following completion of each of the steps previously described, and in partnership with Nurse Coaching experts and endorsing organizations, *Professional Nurse Coach Core Curriculum* will be developed and published.

Background Summary

The Art and Science of Nurse Coaching brings one dimension of nursing's leadership role in healthcare reform to the forefront. This document will also assist nurses involved in interprofessional conversations related to the establishment of standards of practice and a credentialing process for health and wellness coaches (Kreitzer, Sierpina, & Lawson, 2008; Lawson, 2009; Moore & Tschannen-Moran, 2010; NCCHWC, 2011).

This document clarifies nursing perspectives concerning the role of the Nurse Coach in five key ways: (1) It specifies the philosophy, beliefs, and values of the Nurse Coach and the Nurse Coach's scope of practice; (2) It articulates the relationship between *The Art and Science of Nurse Coaching* and *Nursing: Scope and Standards of Practice,* 2nd Edition (ANA, 2010a); (3) It provides the basis for continued interdisciplinary conversations related to professional health and wellness coaches and lay health and wellness coaches; (4) It lays the foundation for an international certification process for professional Nurse Coaching practice; and (5) It identifies the need to develop a core curriculum for professional Nurse Coaching practice that can be used in practice, education, research, and healthcare policy.

Appendix A. The Art and Science of Nurse Coaching, 1st Edition

Appendix B.

The American Holistic Nurses Credentialing Corporation (AHNCC) Nurse Coach Certification Process

Initiating Nursing Alliances

The PNCW entered into a conversation with the American Holistic Nurse Credentialing Corporation (AHNCC) regarding the paradigm shift toward health and wellness inherent in the Patient Protection and Affordable Care Act, and the importance of developing a role and certification program for the professional Nurse Coach. Given that holistic nurses specialize in the practice of health and wellness, it was mutually determined that AHNCC was the appropriate venue for a national certification program for professional Nurse Coaches. After lengthy discussion, the PNCW entered an agreement with AHNCC whereby AHNCC would sponsor the work of the PNCW in exchange for the rights to establish a national certification process for the Nurse Coach.

Certification Examination Development

AHNCC and the Professional Testing Corporation of New York (PTC) collaborated to develop a set of competencies extrapolated from the literature and in accordance with *Nursing: Scope and Standards of Practice*, 2nd ed. (ANA, 2010a). The competencies, reviewed by three expert panels, were revised until approved, and then used for a role-delineation study. The results from that role-delineation study were used to develop a Blueprint, and guide the development of the Nurse Coach certification examination.

A multiple-step process, overseen by PTC, was used to develop the examination including: item-writing to assess specified competencies, item-reviews to assess content validity, and an exam-development process to assess content and construct validity. An item-analysis step, to assess for reliability, is undertaken following the administration of each examination. The Nurse Coach examination will be piloted February, 2013. Additional information is available on the AHNCC website: www.ahncc.org or http://www.ahncc.org/certification/nursecoachnchwnc.html.

Appendix C.

The Nurse Coach Role in Healthcare Transformation

Appendix C documents the forces that catalyzed the initial grassroots work of six nurses to create this document and describes how the professional Nurse Coach role can contribute to national and global healthcare transformation.

Nurse Coaches in National Healthcare Transformation

Nurse Coaches can be leaders in engaging clients in self-care and adoption of healthy life style behaviors that lead to improved healthcare outcomes. A focus on transformation of health care is leading to new models of care delivery that incorporate the professional Nurse Coach role. In 23 of the 24 models discussed in *Innovative Care Delivery Models: Identifying New Models that Effectively Leverage Nurses* (Kimball, Joynt, Cherner, & ONeill, 2007), organizations created new roles for nurses that gave increased accountability for achieving successful patient quality, safety, and satisfaction outcomes. The concept of Nurse Coaches was also described as helping patients make successful transitions across settings.

In 2008, the Samueli Institute released its visionary report entitled *Wellness Initiative for the Nation (WIN)* (2008). This report advocated new approaches to health prevention and health promotion. Referring to a "broken disease treatment system" (p. 4), the authors stated that a new vision of health based upon human flourishing is needed. The report presented the idea of health coaches as one way to significantly reduce healthcare costs and mortality. They and others realized that current healthcare delivery practices, whether conventional or holistic, are in need of models of care that provide a wide range of choices for individuals that are efficient, effective, and reduce costs. This is fundamental to transforming health care from a disease-based model of care to one that focuses on health and wellness.

In March 2010, the Patient Protection and Affordable Care Act (PPACA) became law (HR3590) (Patient Protection and Affordable Care Act, 2010). The language in the PPACA refers to partnerships with a diverse group of licensed health professionals including practitioners of integrative health, preventive medicine, health coaching, public education, and more.

Many provisions in health care home and accountable care models are based on interprofessional care coordination that is patient-centered. The Agency for Healthcare Research and Quality (AHRQ) has funded and published projects that clearly address the need for a revitalized care system where decisions are based within the context of patient's values and preferences (Meyers et al., 2010). Asking patients and families what matters most to them is a critical step in engaging them in care. Coordinated patient-centered care that includes actively engaged patients requires a new set of skills for providers, patients, and families (Scholle, Torda, Peikes, Han, & Genevro, 2010).

In December 2010, the Healthy People 2020 initiative (U.S. Department of Health and Human Services, n.d.) was announced. This exhaustive, multiyear, collaborative process among the U.S. Department of Health and Human Services (HHS) and other federal agencies, public stakeholders, and the advisory committee continues the work started in 2000 with the Healthy People 2010 plan for improving the nation's health. (See also the discussion of Healthy People 2020 on pages 23 and 29.)

In June 2011, the National Prevention, Health Promotion, and Public Health Council announced the release of the National Prevention and Health Promotion Strategy, a comprehensive plan that will help increase the number of Americans who are healthy at every stage of life (National Prevention Strategy, 2011). The National Prevention and Health Promotion Strategy document addresses the importance of healthy foods, clean air and water, and safe worksites that is directly related to national and global healthcare transformation. (See also the discussion of the National Prevention Strategy in this document.)

Professional Nurse Coaches and Global Healthcare Transformation

To achieve global healthcare transformation, the United Nations Millennium Development Goals (MDGs), declared in 2000, must be achieved for the 21st century to progress toward a sustainable quality of life for all of humanity (United Nations, 2011). These eight MDGs are as follows:

- MDG 1. Eradicate Extreme Poverty and Hunger

- MDG 2. Achieve Universal Primary Education

- MDG 3. Promote Gender Equality and Empower Women

- MDG 4. Reduce Child Mortality

- MDG 5. Improve Maternal Health

- MDG 6. Combat HIV/AIDS

- MDG 7. Ensure Environmental Sustainability

- MDG 8. Develop Global Partnerships

These Goals are an ambitious agenda for improving lives worldwide. Of these eight, MDGs 4, 5, and 6 are directly related to health and nursing. The other five (MDGs 1, 2, 3, 7, and 8) are factors that determine the health or lack of health of people. For each goal, one target to be achieved by 2015 has been established, using 1990 data as a benchmark.

"Health" is the common thread that runs through all eight UN MDGs. Professional Nurse Coaches are part of the 17.6 million nurses and midwives of the world (WHO, 2009). They understand that these goals point directly back to the work Florence Nightingale achieved in her time (Nightingale Declaration for a Healthy World, n.d.). These goals are directly related to the work of all nurses everywhere, many of whom who are engaged in coaching people to find local solutions at the global level.

The leadership of professional Nurse Coaches can initiate new approaches to improved global health by empowering individuals and groups to carry Nightingale's legacy forward into the 21st century to address the environmental and social determinates of health. New efforts must be implemented to prevent disease and to create strategies for a healthy and fit world, recognizing that prevention must become part of daily life. This is the work of the four international organizations discussed next.

International Council of Nurses

The International Council of Nurses (ICN) is a federation of more than 130 national nurses associations that represent the millions of nurses worldwide (ICN, n.d.). Founded in 1899, ICN is the world's first and widest reaching international organization for health professionals. Operated by nurses, ICN works to ensure the quality of nursing care for all, sound health policies globally, the advancement of nursing knowledge, and the presence worldwide of a respected nursing profession and a competent and satisfied nursing workforce. Professional Nurse Coaches can contribute to the quality of nursing care, influence healthcare policy, and be involved in scientific advances.

Global Network of WHO Collaborating Centres for Nursing and Midwifery Development

To organize nursing and midwifery leadership, the Global Network of WHO Collaborating Centres (WHOCCs) for Nursing and Midwifery Development is an independent, international, non-for-profit, voluntary organization, currently comprising 44 institutions of excellence, from the six regions of the World Health Organization (WHO) (WHOCC, n.d.). Founded in 1988, the Network strives to enhance the collaborative activities of Nursing and Midwifery Collaborating Centres, supporting WHO's efforts towards Health for All (World Health Organization, 2011). Professional Nurse Coaches can include coaching skills in the provision of direct care. They can also advocate for the UN's MDG4 (Reduce Child Mortality), which is related to the health of infants. MDG 5 (Improve Maternal Health) sits at the core of one of today's most critical global health concerns. Clearly nursing practice has been and must continue to be integrally involved in this challenge.

CGFNS International

CGFNS International (also known as the Commission on Graduates of Foreign Nursing Schools) is to serve the global community through programs and services that verify and promote the knowledge-based practice competency of healthcare professionals. The Commission on Graduates for Foreign Nursing Schools (CGFNS) began in 1977. CGFNS has reviewed and/or certified the credentials of over 500,000 foreign-educated nurses and other healthcare professionals for U.S. licensure and immigration. The vision of CGFNS is to be the premier source of credentials evaluation and professional development services that provide strategic value and direction to healthcare professionals worldwide (CGFNS, n.d.). The Nurse Coach recognizes the importance of sound credentialing and deepening the professional development of the nurse.

Sigma Theta Tau International

The Honor Society of Nursing, Sigma Theta Tau International (STTI), founded in 1922 with 125,000 active members, has as its mission to support the learning, knowledge and professional development of nurses committed to making a difference in health worldwide (STTI, n.d.). The STTI vision is to create a global community of nurses who lead in using knowledge, scholarship, service and learning to improve the health of the world's people. The importance of the professional Nurse Coach role has been recognized by STTI, as evidenced by the organization's publication of *Coaching in Nursing* (Donner & Wheeler, 2009).

Appendix A. The Art and Science of Nurse Coaching, 1st Edition

Appendix D.

Theories in Nurse Coaching Practice

Overview: Nursing Theories and Other Theories

Appendix D provides an overview of the recognized meta-paradigm in nursing and patterns of knowing with application to professional Nurse Coaching. It also discusses many frequently used nursing theories and other social theories in professional Nurse Coaching practice. The nursing theories discussed are Rogers' Theory of Science of Unitary Human Beings, Orem's Self-Care Deficit Nursing Theory, Roy's Adaptation Model, Neuman's Systems Model, Parse's Theory of Human Becoming, Barrett's Knowing Participation in Change Theory, Erickson's Theory of Modeling and Role-Modeling, Watson's Theory of Human Science and Human Care, Newman's Health as Expanding Consciousness Theory, and Dossey's Theory of Integral Nursing. Social science and other theories and concepts that are often used in Nurse Coaching include change theories, positive psychology, resilience, coherence theory, complexity science, energy theories, story theory, and reflective practice.

Nursing Meta-Paradigm and Patterns of Knowing and Its Application to Professional Nurse Coaches

Paradigms and worldviews can impact Nurse Coaches as they reflect on the nature of human beings, health, environment, and caring. Fawcett (1995) articulated four components recognized as the meta-paradigm in a nurse theory—nurse, person, health, and environment (society). Meta-paradigm definitions may vary in different nursing theories; however, the four domains are seen as interrelated and interdependent and each informs and influences the others.

As a way to organize nursing knowledge, Carper (Carper, 1978) in her now classic 1978 article, identified the four fundamental patterns of knowing (personal, empirics, ethics, aesthetics) followed by Munhall's (1993) introduction of the pattern of not knowing, and White's (1995) introduction of the pattern of sociopolitical knowing. These patterns continue to be refined and reframed with new applications and interpretations. Understanding these patterns of knowing can assist Nurse Coaches to bring themselves into the full expression of being present in the moment with self and others, to integrate aesthetics with science, and to develop the flow of ethical experience with thinking and acting.

Nursing Theories

Theory of Science of Unitary Human Beings

Martha Rogers (1970, 1994) was one of the first contemporary nurse scholars to articulate the idea that humans are whole beings and cannot be understood by reducing them to parts. "The descriptive, explanatory, and predictive principles that direct professional nursing practice are rooted in a fundamental concept of the wholeness of life" (Rogers, 1970, p. 34.) Her ideas, developed over several years, led to the development of the Science of Unitary Human Beings. Rogers' ideas encompassed a pan-dimensional and transcendent view of humans as ever evolving energy fields. Rogers encouraged nurses not to become stuck in present reality, but to look forward to envision how life might be in a universe where there is continuous change (Rogers, 1994).

Self-Care Deficit Nursing Theory

Dorothea Orem's Self-Care Deficit Nursing Theory (SCDNT) was first published in 1971 and subsequently expanded through 2001 (Orem, 1971, Hartweg & Fleck, 2009). She saw people as individuals that should be self-reliant and responsible for their own care. Self-care and dependent care are behaviors that are learned within a socio-political context. A person's knowledge related to health and potential health problems is necessary to promote self-care behaviors. Nursing is a form of action and interaction between two or more individuals. Successfully meeting universal and development self-care requisites is an important component of primary care prevention. She defined self-care as the practice of activities that individuals initiate and perform to maintain life, health and well-being. Self-care agency implies a person's ability for engaging in self-care conditioned by age developmental state, life experiences, sociocultural orientation and available resources. Therapeutic self-care demand is described as the totality of self-care actions to be performed for some duration to meet the person's self-care requisites. Self-care requisites are any actions directed towards provision of self-care. Nursing is required when an individual (dependent) is unable or limited in the ability to provide continuous and effective care.

Adaption Model
Sister Callista Roy's (2009) model appeared in 1970 with an expansion in the mid-70s to the mid-80s. The Adaption Model major concepts include people as adaptive systems (both individuals and groups), environment, health, and the goal of nursing using the six-step nursing process. She views the individual as a set of interrelated, biological, psychological, and social systems. She believes that all individuals strive to maintain balance and cope with life's challenges, with each person having a unique style. It is this individual range of adaptability that determines how one deals with new experiences and challenges. There are four main adaptation systems: (1) the physiological-physical system, (2) the self-concept group identity system, (3) the role mastery/function system, and (4) the interdependency system. Roy's goal of nursing is the promotion of adaptation in each of the four modes that contribute to the individual's health, quality of life, and dignity in dying. Roy sees the person as a bio-psychosocial being constantly interacting with a changing environment. The person is an open system who uses coping skills to deal with life's problems and challenges. Health is the process of being and becoming an integrated and whole person. The environment is seen as all conditions and behaviors of the person. It is a universal model adaptable to numerous situations. The nurse's role is to promote system stability by using three levels of prevention.

Neuman Systems Model
Betty Neuman (Neuman & Fawcett, 2010) developed the Neuman Systems Model (NSM) in 1970 and was first published in 1974. She replaced the word *patient* with the word *client*. She views the client as a holistic being which physiological, psychological, sociological, and developmental aspects. This model is based on the client's relationship to stress, reaction to it, and reconstitution factors that are dynamic and changing.

Theory of Human Becoming

Rosemarie Rizzo Parse (1981, 1995) developed the idea of the person as a unitary whole suggesting that the person can only be viewed as a unity. She describes nursing as a scientific discipline and the practice of nursing as an art in which nurses serve as guides to assist others in making choices affecting health. Person is a unified, whole being. Health is a process of becoming; it is a personal commitment, an unfolding, a process related to lived experiences. Environment is the universe. The human-universe is inseparable and evolving as one. The concept of "presence" is emphasized in this theory as a critically important nurse intervention.

Knowing Participation in Change Theory

Elisabeth Barrett (1983, 1989, 2003) developed the Knowing Participation in Change Theory. Her power theory elaborates on Martha Rogers' (1970) axiom that humans can participate knowingly in change. She proposed that power is the capacity to participate knowingly in the nature of change characterizing the continuous mutual process of people and their world. Power as knowing participation in change is being aware of what one is choosing to do, feeling free to do it, and doing it intentionally. According to this theory, power is inherently value free. The observable, measurable dimensions of power are awareness, choices, freedom to act intentionally, and involvement in creating change. The inseparable association of the four power dimensions is termed a person's or group's Power Profile. The Power Profile is not static; it varies based on the changing nature of the human-environment mutual process of various individuals and/or groups. These changes indicate: (1) the nature of the awareness of experiences; (2) the type of choices made; (3) the degree to which freedom to act intentionally is operating; and (4) the manner of involvement in creating specific changes.

Modeling and Role-Modeling Theory

Helen Erickson and her colleagues (Erickson, Tomlin, & Swain, 1983/2009) published a theory and paradigm for nursing called the Modeling and Role-Modeling Theory that draws on work from many theoretical perspectives. In this theory there are five aims of all nursing interventions: (1) to build trust; (2) to promote positive orientation; (3) to promote perceived control; (4) to promote strengths; and (5) to set mutual goals that are health-directed. The nurse uses this theory by creating a model of the client's world (*Modeling*) and then uses that model to plan interventions and to demonstrate and support health-producing behaviors from within the client's worldview (*Role Modeling*). This theory depicts nursing as a process that demands an interpersonal and interactive relationship with the client. Facilitation, nurturance, and unconditional acceptance must characterize the nurse's care giving. The human person is seen as a holistic being with interacting subsystems (biologic, psychological, social, and cognitive), and with an inherent genetic base and spiritual drive; the whole is greater than the sum of its parts (Erickson, 2010).

Theory of Human Science and Human Care

Jean Watson (1985, 2007) emphasizes the relationship between two beings as fundamental for nursing practice: it must never be diminished or lost. Nursing's role in society is based on human caring. Caring is our moral imperative. Caring and loving are primal energetic forces; we all need to be loved and cared for. Transpersonal caring is a means of moving toward a higher sense of self and harmony with mind, body, and soul. Access to a higher sense of self is accessed through one's emotions and thoughts—the subjective inner world. Transpersonal caring allows humanity to grow towards greater harmony, spiritual evolution, and perfection. The transpersonal caring relationship depends upon: (1) a moral commitment to human dignity; (2) the nurse's intent and will to affirm the subjective significance of other; (3) the nurse's ability to detect feelings; (4) the nurse's ability to feel a union with another; and (5) the nurse's own history.

Health as Expanding Consciousness Theory

Margaret Newman (1986, 1994) describes health as the expansion of consciousness. The theory of Health as Expanded Consciousness is grounded in Newman's personal experience and was stimulated by Rogers' (1970) description of the unitary nature of a human being in interaction with the environment. Health and illness is a single process moving through varying degrees of organization and disorganization, but all one unitary process. The total pattern of person-environment is a network of consciousness. Consciousness is everywhere. A person, rather than possessing consciousness, *is* consciousness. Consciousness is ever evolving, and "the process of evolution of consciousness is also the process of health" (Newman, 1986, p. 43). In Newman's model of health, there is no basis for rejecting any experience as irrelevant. The important factor is to become attuned to one's pattern of interaction and to recognize that it is one of expanding consciousness. The nurse practicing from this understanding "enters into a partnership with the client with the mutual goal of participating in an authentic relationship, trusting that in the process of evolving, both will grow and become healthier in the sense of higher levels of consciousness" (p. 68).

Theory of Integral Nursing

Barbara Dossey (2009, 2013) has developed her Theory of Integral Nursing, which includes an integral worldview and four perspectives of human experience and reality: (1) the individual interior; (2) the individual exterior; (3) the collective interior; and (4) the collective exterior. Each perspective is considered equally important. The Theory of Integral Nursing builds upon a solid holistic, integrated, and multidimensional theoretical nursing foundation and may be used with other integral and holistic nursing concepts, theories, and research. The integral approach allows nurses to more fully consider and comprehend the complexity of human experience. Healing is a core concept of the Theory of Integral Nursing. Healing is "the innate natural phenomenon that comes from within a person and describes the indivisible wholeness and the interconnectedness of all people, and all things" (Dossey, 2013, p. 27).

Change Theories

Behavioral change theories most frequently used in professional Nurse Coaching include the Transtheoretical Stages of Change Model (Prochaska, Norcross, & DeClemente, 1995), the Health Belief Model (Becker, 1990), Self-Efficacy (Bandura, 1977), Immunity to Change (Kegan & Lahey, 2009), and Motivational Interviewing (Dart, 2011; Miller & Rollnick, 2002; Rollnick, Miller, & Butler, 2008) and have been adopted by many Nurse Coaches (Hess et al., 2010). Concepts and strategies embedded within these approaches are applied in coaching interactions to promote self-efficacy and to uncover resistance and identify barriers to change. Appreciative Inquiry (Cooperrider & Whitney, 2005; Cooperrider, Whitney, & Stavros, 2005; Moore & Charvat, 2007) is another model of change that focuses on client strengths to create a more positive future, while Unitary Appreciative Inquiry (Cowling, 2001) is a related approach utilized by nurses to know the wholeness and uniqueness of each person as the context for change.

Positive Psychology

Positive psychology is a recent branch of psychology that places emphasis on ways to make normal life more fulfilling and focuses on strengths and human flourishing (Seligman, 1990; Csikszentmihalyi, 1990). Researchers study states of flow, values, strengths, virtues and talents and how these areas can be enhanced in social systems, organizations, and institutions. This field does not replace traditional psychology. At the *subjective level* the focus is on the positive subjective experience, which includes: well-being and satisfaction (past), and flow, joy, the sensual pleasures, and happiness (present), and constructive cognitions about the future-optimism, hope, and faith. At the *individual level* it is about positive individual traits: the capacity for love and vocation, courage, interpersonal skill, aesthetic sensibility, perseverance, forgiveness, originality, future-mindedness, high talent, and wisdom. At the *group level* it is about the civic virtues and the institutions that move individuals toward better citizenship: responsibility, nurturance, altruism, civility, moderation, tolerance, and work ethic.

Resilience

Resilience is generally considered to be a positive trait involving the capacity to cope with stress and adversity (McCraty & Childers, 2010). Resilience can be an outcome of good coaching and emerges from learned optimism (Seligman, 1990). *Physical resilience* is reflected in physical flexibility, endurance, and strength. *Mental resilience* is reflected in one's attention span, mental flexibility, optimistic worldview, and ability to integrate multiple points of view. *Emotional resilience* is related to one's ability to self-regulate the expression of one's emotions. *Spiritual resilience* is related to one's commitment to one's core values, the ability to trust one's intuition, and tolerance of others' values and beliefs. While questions remain concerning the development of resilience (Atkinson, Martin, & Rankin, 2009), there are nurse scholars who contend that development of resilience is a process that can be supported and developed at any time, and that development of resilience has the potential to improve clinical outcomes (Gillespie, Chaboyer, & Wallis, 2007; Warelow, 2005).

Sense-of-Coherence Theory

The Sense-of-Coherence (SOC) theory is a theory of salutogenesis. Developed by Antonovsky (1996), this theory represents a perspective that is different from a traditional pathogenic orientation of health. The focus is on what makes a person move towards health. "The focus is on the story of the person rather than the diagnosis. The person is understood as an open system in active interaction with the environment (both external and internal conditions)" (Langeland, Wahl, Kristoffersen, & Hanestad, 2007, p. 277). A sense of coherence concerns the extent to which one has a feeling of confidence that one's internal and external environments are predictable and can be explained. The Sense-of-Coherence theory contains three components: comprehensibility, manageability, and meaningfulness. Comprehensibility refers to the ability to understand situations. Manageability refers to a person's perception that needed resources are available. Meaningfulness refers to the extent to which life is perceived as making sense emotionally and is often considered the most important component (Langeland, et al, 2007). A sense of coherence will influence the motivation to engage in self-management of one's health (Chenworth, Gallagher, Sheriff, Donoghue, & Stein-Parbury, 2008).

Complexity Science

Quantum or complexity science is a set of theoretical constructs that look at the universe as comprised of complex adaptive systems – as a set of interrelationships (Malloch & Porter-O'Grady, 2005). All is connected. Relationships between and among individuals and their collective relationships to systems create a complex whole. Change is achieved through small and successful increments that when aggregated lead to greater and broader change. The nonlinearity of complex adaptive systems favors continuous innovation and creativity over stability, strict formats, and unchanging structures. Nurses who can adapt and co-evolve with new situations as they emerge—who are able to focus on process, avoiding rigid goals and prescriptive content (Wilson, 2009)— are maximally positioned to be change facilitators. In quantum change, all process is dynamic and continuous; it neither begins nor ends. One moves in dance as conditions adapt and change, and change again. Underneath surface appearances lie chaos, unpredictability, paradox, and complexity—foundations upon which new order and symmetry will appear.

Reflective Practice

Reflective practice is the process of developing new insights through self-awareness and critical reflection upon experiences – both past experiences and in-the-moment experiences (Freshwater, Taylor, & Sherwood, 2008). Reflective nursing practice involves the capacity to be open to different viewpoints and to recognize opportunities for change. "Being mindful is the quintessential nature of reflective practice" (Johns, 2010, p. 313). Being mindful involves being a witness without judgment; it transcends the rational mind and integrates all knowing.

Appendix A. The Art and Science of Nurse Coaching, 1st Edition

212 • The Art and Science of Nurse Coaching, 2nd Ed. • Appendix A

Appendix E.

Interventions Frequently Used in Nurse Coaching Practice

Many of these interventions are listed in the current Nursing Interventions Classification system (NIC, n.d.).

- Affirmation
- Appreciative Inquiry
- Aromatherapy
- Art Therapy
- Celebration
- Client Assessments
- Cognitive Reframing
- Contracts
- Deep Listening
- Exercise
- Goal Setting
- Guided Imagery
- Holistic Self-Assessments
- Humor and Laughter
- Intention
- Journaling
- Meditation
- Mindfulness Practice

- Motivational Interviewing
- Movement
- Music and Sound Therapy
- Observation
- Play
- Powerful Questions
- Prayer
- Presence
- Probing Questions
- Reflection
- Relaxation Modalities
- Ritual
- Self-Care Interventions
- Self-Reflection
- Silence
- Somatic Awareness
- Stories
- Visioning

Appendix B
Metaparadigm in Nursing and Selected Nurse Theorists that Align with Professional Nurse Coaching Practice

Appendix B provides an overview of the recognized metaparadigm in nursing, patterns of knowing in nursing, and the nurse theorists that most align with nurse coaching practice, education, research, and healthcare policy.

Metaparadigm in Nursing

Nurse Coaches expand their paradigms and worldviews as they reflect on the nature of human beings, health, environment, and caring. Fawcett (1995) articulated four components recognized as the metaparadigm in a nurse theory—nurse, person, health, and environment (society). Metaparadigm definitions may vary in different nursing theories; however, the four domains are seen as interrelated and interdependent and each informs and influences the others. *Note.* Nurse coaching metaparadigm description details are found in the Philosophical Principles of Professional Nurse Coaching section.

Patterns of Knowing in Nursing

As a way to organize nursing knowledge, Carper (1978) in her now classic 1978 article, identified the four fundamental patterns of knowing (personal, empirics, ethics, aesthetics) followed by Munhall's (1993) introduction of the pattern of not knowing, and White's (1995) introduction of the pattern of sociopolitical knowing. These patterns continue to be refined and reframed with new applications and interpretations. Nurse coaches are expanding their understanding of these patterns of knowing to bring themselves into the full expression of being present in the moment with self and others, to integrate aesthetics with science, and to develop the flow of ethical experience with thinking and acting. These patterns of knowing in nursing are described next (Dossey, 2016).

Personal Knowing. The nurse's dynamic process and awareness of wholeness that focuses on the synthesis of perceptions and being with self. It may be developed through art, meditation, dance, music, stories, and other expressions of the authentic and genuine self in daily life and nursing practice. This may be related to living and nonliving people and things, such as a deceased relative, animal, or a lost precious object through flashes of memories stimulated by a current situation (a touch may bring forth past memories of abuse or suffering). Insights may be gained through dreams and other reflective practices that reveal symbols, images, and other connections that also influence one's interior environment.

Empirical Knowing. The science of nursing that focuses on formal expression, replication, and validation of scientific competence in nursing education and practice. It is expressed in models and theories and can be integrated into evidence-based practice. Empirical indicators are accessed through the known senses that are subject to direct observation, measurement, and verification.

Aesthetic Knowing. The art of nursing that focuses on how to explore experiences and meaning in life with self or another that includes authentic presence, the nurse as a facilitator of healing, and the artfulness of a healing environment. It is the combination of knowledge, experience, instinct, and intuition that connects the nurse with a patient or client in order to explore the meaning of a situation about the human experiences of life, health, illness, and death. It calls forth resources and inner strengths from the nurse to be a facilitator in the healing process. It is the integration and expression of all the other patterns of knowing in nursing praxis.

Ethical Knowing. The moral knowledge in nursing that focuses on behaviors, expressions, and dimensions of both morality and ethics. It includes valuing and clarifying situations to create formal moral and ethical behaviors intersecting with legally prescribed duties. It emphasizes respect for the person, the family, and the community that encourages connectedness and relationships that enhance attentiveness, responsiveness, communication, and moral action.

Not Knowing. The capacity to use healing presence, to be open spontaneously to the moment with no preconceived answers or goals to be obtained. It engages authenticity, mindfulness, openness, receptivity, surprise, mystery, and discovery with self and others in the subjective space and the intersubjective space that allows for new solutions, possibilities, and insights to emerge. It acknowledges the patterns that may not be understood that may manifest related to various situations or relationships.

Sociopolitical Knowing. The important contextual variables of social, economic, geographic, cultural, political, historical, and other key factors in theoretical, evidence-based practice and research. This pattern includes informed critique and social justice for the voices of the underserved in all areas of society along with protocols to reduce health disparities.

Selected Nurse Theorists Most Aligned With Nurse Coaching

The nursing theorists and their theories most aligned with nurse coaching are listed in order of the first publication and are discussed in four different categories as follows:

- Conceptual Models/Grand Theories in the Integrative–Interactive Paradigm
- Conceptual Models and Grand Theories in the Unitary–Transformative Paradigm
- Grand Theories about Care or Caring Paradigm
- Middle-Range Theories

Conceptual Models/Grand Theories in the Integrative–Interactive Paradigm

Sister Callista Roy—Roy Adaption Model (RAM). Roy's (Roy, 2009) model was first published in 1970 with an expansion in the mid-70s to the mid-80s. The RAM major concepts include people as adaptive systems (both individuals and groups), the environment, health, and the goal of nursing using the six-step nursing process. Roy views the individual as a set of interrelated systems, biological, psychological, and social. She believes that all individuals strive to maintain balance and cope with life's challenges with each person having a unique style. It is this individual range of adaptability that determines how one deals with new experiences and challenges. There are four main adaptation systems as follows: 1) the physiological-physical system; 2) the self-concept group identity system; 3) the role mastery/function system; and 4) the inter-dependency system. Roy sees the person as a bio-psychosocial being constantly interacting with a changing environment. The person is an open system who uses coping skills to deal with life's problems and challenges. Health is the process of being and becoming an integrated and whole person. The environment is seen as all conditions and behaviors of the person. Roy's goal of nursing is the promotion of adaptation in each of the four modes that contribute to the individual's health, quality of life, and dignity in dying.

Betty Neuman—Neuman Systems Model (NSM). Neuman's (Neuman & Fawcett, 2010) model was developed in 1970 and first published in 1974. The NSM uses the word client instead of patient. She views the client as a holistic being that includes the physiological, psychological, sociological, and developmental aspects. This model is based on the client's relationship to stress, reaction to it, and the reconstitution factors that are dynamic and changing. It is considered universal in nature that allows its adaptability. The NSM central philosophy consists of energy resources that are surrounded by three things: several lines of resistance, which represent the internal factors helping the client fight against a stressor; the normal line of defense, which represents the patient's equilibrium; and the flexible line of defense, which represents the dynamic nature that can rapidly change over a short time. The nurse's role is to keep the system's stability by using three levels of prevention. The first is primary prevention, which protects the normal line and strengthens the flexible line of defense. The secondary prevention is used to strengthen the internal lines of resistance, which reduces the reaction and increases resistance factors. Finally, tertiary prevention readapts, stabilizes, and protects the patient's return to wellness after treatment.

Dorothea Orem—Self-Care Deficit Nursing Theory (SCDNT). Orem's (Orem, 1971; Hartweg, 2014) theory was first published in 1971 and subsequently expanded through 2001. The SCDNT views people as individuals that should be self-reliant and responsible for their own care. Self-care and dependent care are behaviors that are learned within a socio-political context. A person's knowledge related to health and potential health problems is necessary to promote self-care behaviors. Nursing is a form of action and interaction between two or more individuals. Successfully meeting universal and development self-care requisites is an important component of primary care prevention and ill health. Orem defined self-care as the practice of activities that individuals initiate and perform to maintain life, health and well-being. Self-care agency implies a person's ability for engaging in self-care that was conditioned by age developmental state, life experiences, sociocultural orientation and available resources. Therapeutic self-care demand is described as the totality of self-care actions to be performed for some duration to meet the person's self-care requisites. Self-care requisites are any action directed towards provision of self-care. Nursing is required when an individual (dependent) is unable or limited in the ability to provide continuous and effective care.

Helen Erickson, Evelyn Tomlin, and Mary Ann Swain—Theory of Modeling and Role Modeling (MRM). Erickson, Tomlin, & Swain's 2009 (Erickson, 2019) theory was first published in 1983 and draws on work from many theoretical perspectives. In this theory there are five aims of all nursing interventions: (1) to build trust; (2) to promote positive orientation; (3) to promote perceived control; (4) to promote strengths; and (5) to set mutual goals that are health-directed. The nurse uses this theory by creating a model of the client's world (Modeling) and then uses that model to plan interventions and to demonstrate and support health-producing behaviors from within the client's worldview (Role Modeling). This theory depicts nursing as a process that demands an interpersonal and interactive relationship with the client. Facilitation, nurturance, and unconditional acceptance must characterize the nurse's care giving. The human person is seen as a holistic being with interacting subsystems (biologic, psychological, social, and cognitive), and with an inherent genetic base and spiritual drive; the whole is greater than the sum of its parts.

Barbara Dossey—Theory of Integral Nursing (TIN). Dossey's (Dossey, 2008; Dossey, 2016; and Dossey, 2020) theory was first published in 2008 and has been expanded. The TIN builds upon a solid holistic, integral, and integrated multidimensional theoretical nursing foundation and may be used with other holistic nursing concepts, theories, and research. Healing is at the core of her theory. She defines healing as the innate natural phenomenon that comes from within a person and describes the indivisible wholeness and the interconnectedness of all people and all things. Her theory also includes the meta-paradigm in nursing, and the patterns of know in nursing. She explores and develops an integral worldview and four integral perspectives of human experience and reality as follows: (1) the individual interior; (2) the individual exterior; (3) the collective interior; and (4) the collective exterior. Each perspective is considered equally important. The integral approach allows nurses to more fully consider and comprehend the complexity of human experience.

Conceptual Models and Grand Theories in the Unitary-Transformative Paradigm

Martha Rogers—Theory of Science of Unitary Human Beings. Rogers' (Rogers, 1970; Rogers, 1994) theory was first published in 1970. She was one of the first contemporary nurse scholars to articulate the idea that humans are whole beings and cannot be understood by reducing them to parts. She viewed the descriptive, explanatory, and predictive principles that direct professional nursing practice as being rooted in a fundamental concept of the wholeness of life. Her ideas, developed over several years, led to the development of the Science of Unitary Human Beings. Rogers' ideas encompassed a pan-dimensional and transcendent view of humans as ever evolving energy fields. Rogers encouraged nurses not to become stuck in present reality, but to look forward and envision how life might be in a universe where there is continuous change.

Rosemarie Rizzo Parse—Theory of Human Becoming. Parse's (Parse, 1995) theory was fist published in 1981. She developed the idea of the person as a unitary whole suggesting that the person can only be viewed as a unity. She describes nursing as a scientific discipline and the practice of nursing as an art in which nurses serve as guides to assist others in making choices affecting health. Person is a unified, whole being. Health is a process of becoming; it is a personal commitment, an unfolding, a process related to lived experiences. Environment is the universe. The human-universe is inseparable and evolving as one. The concept of "presence" is emphasized in this theory as a critically important nurse intervention.

Margaret Newman—Health as Expanding Consciousness Theory. Newman's (Newman, 1994) theory was first published in 1986 and describes health as the expansion of consciousness. The theory of Health as Expanded Consciousness is grounded in Newman's personal experience and was stimulated by Rogers' description of the unitary nature of a human being in interaction with the environment. Health and illness is a single process moving through varying degrees of organization and disorganization, but are all one unitary process. The total pattern of person-environment is a network of consciousness. Consciousness is everywhere. A person, rather than possessing consciousness, is consciousness. She saw consciousness as ever evolving, and this process of evolution of consciousness is also the process of health; there is no basis for rejecting any experience as irrelevant. The important factor is to become attuned to one's pattern of interaction and to recognize that it is one of expanding consciousness. She believed that the nurse practicing from this understanding enters into a partnership with the client with the mutual goal of participating in an authentic relationship, trusting that in the process of evolving, both will grow and become healthier in the sense of higher levels of consciousness.

Richard Cowling—Unitary Knowing in Nursing Practice. Cowling's (Cowling, 2000) theory was first published in 1993. He has further elaborated on the unitary knowing perspective, which was derived from using the science of unitary human beings in practice and considering phenomena within a unitary picture of reality. The systems perspective and the unitary perspective are contrasted as structures for understanding human phenomena in the realm of practice. A model of practice is offered which encompasses the use of experience, perceptions, and expressions as the source of pattern information. The features of unitary knowing involving construction and derivation are presented within the context of unitary pattern nursing.

Grand Theories about Care or Caring Paradigm

Madeleine Leininger—Theory of Transcultural Nursing. Leininger's (Leininger, 2002) theory was first published in 1970 and is based on her ideas of care that contain a strong cultural anthropologic framework. Leininger encouraged nurses to conduct a holistic "culturalological" assessment in the major areas of worldview and social structure factors, including cultural values, beliefs, and practices; religious, philosophical, or spiritual beliefs; economic factors; and educational beliefs. She believed that care was the dominant focus of nursing, which needed a cultural environmental context to be understood and used to ultimately influence nursing care and patient-centered care. A major feature of her theory is the emphasis on the way individuals relate to health, wellbeing, illness, and death in different contexts and cultures. She defined a cultural assessment as a systematic appraisal of individuals, groups, and communities about their cultural beliefs, values, and practices, in order to determine explicit needs within the context of the people being served.

Jean Watson—Theory of Transpersonal Caring/Unitary Caring Science. Watson's (Watson, 2007) original theory was first published in 1979 and expanded over the years. The *Handbook of Caring Science* (Rosa, Horton-Deutsch, & Watson, 2019) compiled the far-reaching impact of her theory in nursing. Watson's emphasizes the relationship between two beings as fundamental for nursing practice: it must never be diminished or lost. Nursing's role in society is based on human caring. Caring is our moral imperative. Caring and loving are primal energetic forces; we all need to be loved and cared for. Transpersonal caring is a means of moving toward a higher sense of self and harmony with mind, body, and soul. Access to a higher sense of self is accessed through one's emotions and thoughts – the subjective inner world. Transpersonal caring allows humanity to grow towards greater harmony, spiritual evolution, and perfection. The transpersonal caring relationship depends upon: (1) a moral commitment to human dignity; (2) the nurse's intent and will to affirm the subjective significance of other; (3) the nurse's ability to detect feelings; (4) the nurse's ability to feel a union with another; and (5) the nurse's own history.

Middle-Range Theories

Hildegard Peplau—Theory of Interpersonal Relations. Hildegard Peplau (1952) created the middle-range nursing theory of interpersonal relations, which helped to revolutionize the scholarly work of nurses. "Peplau's theory focuses on the phases of the interpersonal process that occur when an ill person and a nurse come together to resolve a health-related difficulty." (Fawcett, J., & DeSanto-Madeya, S. (2013). Peplau's major concepts, include nursing, person, health, and environment and the process to better understand nurse-patient interactive phenomena.

Elisabeth Barrett—Knowing Participation in Change Theory. Barrett's (Barrett, 2003) theory was first published in 1983 and elaborates on Martha Rogers' (Rogers, 1970) axiom that humans can participate knowingly in change (Barrett, 1983). She proposed that power is the capacity to participate knowingly in the nature of change characterizing the continuous mutual process of people and their world. Power as knowing participation in change is being aware of what one is choosing to do, feeling free to do it, and doing it intentionally. According to this theory, power is inherently value free. The observable, measurable dimensions of power are awareness, choices, freedom to act intentionally, and involvement in creating change. The inseparable association of the four power dimensions is termed a person's or group's Power Profile. The Power Profile is not static; it varies based on the changing nature of the human-environment mutual process of various individuals and groups. These changes indicate: 1) the nature of the awareness of experiences; 2) the type of choices made; 3) the degree to which freedom to act intentionally is operating; and 4) the manner of involvement in creating specific changes.

Merle H. Mishel—Theory of Uncertainty in Illness (UIT). Mishel's (Mishel, 1988; Clayton, Dean, & Mishel, 2018) theory was first published in 1988 and further expanded. The UIT proposes that uncertainty exists in illness situations that are ambiguous, complex, unpredictable, and when information is unavailable or inconsistent. Uncertainty is defined as the inability to determine the meaning of illness-related events. It is a cognitive state created when the individual cannot adequately structure or categorize an illness event because of insufficient cues. The reconceptualized theory of uncertainty (RUIT) retains the definitions to uncertainty and major themes but adds the concepts of self-organization and probabilistic thinking (Michel, 1990). This theory assists to support clients and can reduce uncertainty directly and indirectly. Individuals unfamiliar with the healthcare environment, organization, and expectations may have higher degrees of uncertainty.

Marlaine Smith—Theory of Unitary Caring. Smith's (Smith, 2019) theory was first published in 1999 following her in depth analysis of the caring literature. This analysis revealed that caring was a multidimensional concept that assumed multiple meanings depending on the framework within which it was situated or the lens from which it was view. Her theory contains five concepts as follows: 1) Manifesting Intentions; 2) Appreciating Pattern; 3) Attuning to Dynamic Flow: 4) Experience the Infinite; and 5) Inviting Creative Emergence.

Mary Jane Smith and Patricia Liehr—Story Theory. Smith and Liehr's (Leihr & Smith, 2018) theory was first published in 1999 and further expanded. It describes story as a narrative happening wherein a person connects with self-in relation through nurse-person intentional dialogue to create ease. Clients' stories infuse bodily responses with unique meaning. Story Theory has seven phases of inquiry as follows: Phase 1: Gather a story about what matters most about a complication health challenge (or current situation); Phase 2: Compose a reconstructed story; Phase 3: Connect existing literature to the health challenge; Phase 4: Refine the name of the complicating challenge; Phase 5: Describe the developing story plot with high points, low points, and turning points; Phase 6: Identify movement towards resolving; and Phase 7: Collect additional stories about the health challenge.

Richard Cowling—Unitary Appreciative Inquiry. Cowling's (Cowling, 2001) theory was first published in 2001. Unitary appreciative inquiry is described as an orientation, a process, and approach for illuminating the wholeness, uniqueness, and essence that is the pattern of human life unitary appreciative inquiry provides a way of giving fullest attention to important facets of human life that are often not fully accounted for in current methods that have a heavier emphasis on diagnostic representations. The critical dimensions of nursing knowledge development expressed in dialectics of the general and the particular, action and theory, stories and numbers, sense and soul, aesthetics and empirics, and interpretation and emancipation are considered in the context of the unitary appreciative stance.

Barbara Resnick—Theory of Self-Efficacy. Resnick's (Resnick, 2018) theory was first published in 2003. She defines self-efficacy as an individual's judgment of his or her capabilities to organize and execute course of action. The theory was derived from social cognitive theory. Self-efficacy and outcome expectations are influenced within the context of reciprocal determinism. The theory supports ways to motivate individuals to participate in health promoting activities. Resnick believes the theory is situation specific. For example, if an individual has a high degree of self-efficacy with regards to diet management, this may or may not generalize to persistence in an exercise program.

Barbara Dossey, Susan Luck, and Bonney Gulino Schaub—Theory of Integrative Nurse Coaching (TINC). Dossey, Luck, and Schaub's (Dossey, 2015) theory was first published in 2015. It focuses on nursing coaching and guides nurse coaching practice, education, research, and healthcare policy (International Nurse Coach Association, n.d). The TINC offers a bridge between grand nursing theories that encompass the fullest range or the most global phenomena in the nursing discipline. It is broad enough to be useful in complex situations and leads to implications for instrument development, theory testing through research, and nursing practice strategies. The TINC philosophy includes healing, the metaparadigm in nursing theory, and the recognized patterns of knowing in nursing. The TINC has five nurse coaching components as follows: (1) Nurse Coach Self-Development (Self-Reflection, Self-Assessment, Self-Evaluation, Self-Care); (2) Integral Perspectives and Change; (3) Integrative Lifestyle Health and Wellbeing; (4) Awareness and Choice; and (5) Listening with HEART (Healing, Energy, Awareness, Resiliency, Transformation). All five components are fully integrated and have equal value.

Appendix C
Social Science Theories that Align with Professional Nurse Coaching Practice

Appreciative Inquiry

Appreciative Inquiry (AI) is a school of thought in change and development which can be used at an organizational or individual level for initiatives of transformation. The model was founded in 2005 at Case Western Reserve University by David Cooperrider and Diana Whitney. It is based on a structured process that looks at what is working versus what is wrong (Whitney & Cooperrider, 2011). The steps of the framework move through four stages:

1. Discovery Stage. The Discovery stage involves the identification and appreciation of best practices and looks at what is working in the situation. This goes against the common tendency of looking at the "problem". It changes the focus to the positive that often facilitates hope and new energy for change.

2. Dream Stage. The Dream stage is next in which a fresh vision emerges based on renewed optimism and opportunity for something new. The question to ask at this juncture is "What are your hopes and dreams for how this situation could be?"

3. Design Stage. After the different idea has taken some form, the *Design stage* focuses on possibilities. "What could really happen here?" is the question for this step.

4. Destiny Stage. The Destiny stage is the last in the framework. This is the time for details to strengthen the plan for change.

Once the change has been made, the process can begin again looking at what is working and progressing through the stages for continuous reflection and improvement. AI has gained popularity and those interested in this way of working with people, have established training and associations to support the work (Whitney & Cooperrider, 2011). This approach fits well with coaching as it is a positive approach to looking at strengths, successes, vision, planning, and evaluation. AI shares some stages with the nursing process that is used in coaching (Assessment, Diagnosis, etc.).

Complexity Science

Complexity science is not a single theory- it encompasses more than one theoretical framework and is highly interdisciplinary, seeking the answers to some fundamental questions about living, adaptable, changeable systems and economic factors (Davidson, Ray, & Turkel, 2011; Turkel & Ray, 2000). Change is achieved through small and successful increments that when aggregated lead to greater and broader change.

In quantum change, all process is dynamic and continuous; it neither begins or ends. Quantum or complexity science is a set of theoretical constructs that look at the universe as complex adaptive systems – as a set of interrelationships (Malloch & Porter-O'Grady, 2005). Relationships between and among individuals and their collective relationships to systems create a complex whole. The nonlinearity of complex adaptive systems favors continuous innovation and creativity over stability, strict formats, and unchanging structures (Hess et al., 2013, pg. 82).

Nurses who can adapt and co-evolve with new situations as they emerge-who are able to focus on process, avoiding rigid goals and prescriptive content are maximally positioned to be change facilitators (Wilson, 2009). Becoming comfortable with uncertainty, and adapting to change are important skills for nurses as the healthcare landscape evolves.

Five Structures of Integral Consciousness

In Jean Gebser's seminal work, entitled *The Ever Present Origin* (1985), he identified the emergence of specific structures of consciousness or ways of knowing throughout history. He pointed out five structures of consciousness or awareness as follows: 1) archaic, 2) magic, 3) mythical, 4) mental-rational, and 5) integral. Each leads to a new way of knowing and structure of consciousness. His in-depth analysis looked at philosophy, poetry, music, visual arts, architecture, psyche, religion, and other natural sciences as a basis for his theory. His 20th century Western examination of consciousness is supported by East Indian texts (the Manduka Upanishads) from over a thousand years.

The benefit and value of his theory are far reaching: we learn how to utilize valuable mental approaches as well as expand our awareness with more subtle ways of knowing. Gebser describes how to map and access these less familiar structures of consciousness including connection with source, the realm of energy and intuition, along with the world of myth, story, and archetypes. He shows how these ways of knowing enrich and inform our lives at every minute and at multiple levels. Together with the mental, these structures of consciousness provide a specific, detailed, relevant, understandable wholeness framework to inform the interactions in the coaching partnership.

Self-Determination Theory

The landmark study on Self-Determination Theory (SDT) was done at the University of Rochester by Richard Ryan and Edward Deci in 2002 (Ryan & Deci, 2002). Psychodynamic and humanistic theories of personality as well as cognitive theories of development inform SDT.

SDT describes an innate and inherent movement toward psychological growth and integration. Because coaching is a process by which individuals can move toward higher levels of well-being and personal growth, understanding SDT is helpful in identifying the underpinnings of personal development. SDT evolved from studies exploring intrinsic motivation which is seen as playing a dominant role in a person's behavior change. It describes how a person can find intrinsic motivation that can fuel a lasting change through three ingredients. According to STD, a person needs to feel supported in making a change. Coaching is known for the partnership approach in which individuals feel as if the coach is right beside him or her, adding that type of support or relatedness that helps the client begin to make small steady steps forward. As this happens, the second essential ingredient of building intrinsic motivation is occurring: confidence or competence.

As the individual progresses toward their goal, progress is identified and felt by the client. The third and necessary step for intrinsic motivation to occur is autonomy which is at the heart of coaching and separates it from an approach where the healthcare provider is the expert. In coaching the client is the driver: the individual is in charge of the change process and empowered as movement toward growth and integration occur. These elements of STD for intrinsic motivation have been tested across cultures, ages, and gender (Ryan & Deci, 2017).

Health Belief Model

Health Belief Model (HBM) is one of the best known and widely used theories about health behavior change models (Becker, 1974). The HBM explores the beliefs people hold about their health problems and how that affects their action to change, prevent, reduce, or eliminate a health condition in the following six areas.:

- Severity. This aspect of the model refers to how serious the person feels that his or her health condition is and its consequences. According to this research, the more serious, the more effort the individual will put into making changes.

- Susceptibility. If an individual feels that he or she is very susceptible to a health issue, the person will work to avoid the condition. HBM considers that the perceived severity and susceptibility combine into a perceived threat. The higher the perceived threat, the more motivated the person will be do avoid or prevent the condition.

- Benefits. If one believes that taking an action will prevent a health condition, the person is more likely to take action to prevent the condition. For instance, if someone believes that living a very sedentary life can lead to multiple health problems, then the person is more likely to take action.

- Barriers. Perceived benefits must outweigh the barriers (cost, risk, inconvenience, etc.) for a person to taking action.

- Modifying variables. This informs one's perceptions about a health issue and includes demographics (age, sex, culture, location, etc.) and psychosocial aspects (personality, social class, etc.).

- Cues to action. According to this model, a trigger is needed for an individual to take action in regard to a health condition. Perhaps the death of a friend who is similar in age might be an event that would spur one into a positive action to improve health.

Self-efficacy was added to the model and refers to the individual's belief of his or her ability to make a change. This perception might stop one from considering attempting change. The person might believe that they will not be able to start or maintain a new healthier habit pattern (Becker, 1974; Carpenter, 2010).

Immunity to Change

Kegan and Lahey (2009) describe a scenario that stops many people from changing: right conflicting values. For example, a mother might want to take better care of herself but she is also driven to take care of her young children and feels that these needs oppose each other. Through a fairly simple and structured process called the immunity map, the creators of this technique help individuals see how the opposing needs can shift into some more helpful relationship. The mother might realize that when she takes care of herself, she is better able to take care of her children, and suddenly she no longer sees those two needs as conflicting.

To accomplish this transition in thinking, they invite clients to use a 4 column worksheet that helps clients explore the following:

1. Commitment: I am committed to the value or the importance of…

2. What I am doing or not doing that prevents my commitment being fully realized

3. Competing value. I also need…

4. *Big Assumption. I assume that…*

Exploration with the Big Assumption is often the turning point and helps an individual diagnose and overcome their resistance to change. This powerful and easy to use framework helps individuals work with commitment, reward, responsibility, and criticism.

Motivational Interviewing

Miller and Rollnick (2002) describe Motivational interviewing (MI) as a communication tool used to augment and facilitate an individual's motivation to change problematic behaviors. MI is used in various healthcare settings as a patient-centered intervention strategy. It seeks to help patients explore and eventually resolve ambivalence in reference to current health behavior as a guide toward health promotion and disease management. Originally developed in the addictions field, MI has successfully been used in public health and other healthcare sectors.

The fundamental premise of MI is that patients are often ambivalent to change and revert to past habits of least resistance, which may not be supportive of a healthy lifestyle. MI-based discussions are nonjudgmental, empathic, and collaborative, with a focus on strength building. MI can be incorporated into fifteen to twenty minute clinical practice conversations and, when done skillfully, gives both parties the sense of having had quality time together (Miller & Rollnick, 2012).

MI is based on four guiding principles known by the acronym RULE:

1. **Resist the righting reflex**. The nurse coach allows the client to direct the course of change to allow for internal recognition of how a behavior may be impeding progress.

2. **Understand and explore the client's motivation**. The nurse coach explores the clients concerns perceptions, and motivations by allowing the client's story to unfold.

3. **Listen with empathy**. The nurse coach is a skilled listener and highlights for the client, the language and descriptors that may be influencing current behavior.

4. **Empower and encourage hope and optimism**. The nurse coach helps the client discover *how* change can happen, honoring and harnessing intrinsic motivation.

Motivational interviewing uses open-ended statements, affirmations, reflections and summary statements. MI proficiency corresponds with the skill based on self-assessed proficiency in the application of key characteristics of MI.

Positive Psychology

Positive psychology began as a domain of psychology in 1998 and is the study of what makes life worth living or how to flourish on many levels such as body, mind, spirit, environmental, relational, personal, institutional, and global (Seligman, 2006). Maslow (1954) was apparently the first to coin the phrase in 1954 in a chapter titled "Toward a Positive Psychology". It has been called the science of happiness and began to be considered worthwhile and substantive in 1998 based on the work of Martin Seligman (2006). His cohorts and cofounders of the movement were Mihaly Csikszentmihalyi, Chrisopher Peterson, and Barbara Fredrikson. It was an extension of the Humanistic Psychology movement in the 1960s that explored at happiness and wellbeing. Positive psychology is seen as balancing out the disease and illness focus of psychology or providing a more whole picture of the human mind and its functioning. The goal is to minimize pathological thoughts or feeling of hopelessness and build an optimism for life. The focus is on positive emotions, traits and institutions as people celebrate their positive traits, emotions, and virtues as well as build or find communities that support healthy connection, communication, and well-being (Seligman & Csikszentmihalyi, 2014).

Kauffman (2006) describes positive psychology as the heart of coaching because coaching can help people live their best life or create their dreams. Coaching does not focus only on the positive part of living but does help people support their innate drive to growth and development. Coaching is driven by the client who selects the goals which most often lead to a life that is better at many levels.

Psychosynthesis

Roberto Assagioli MD (1888–1974) developed psychosynthesis as a psychological approach to spiritual development (Assagioli, 1965; 1974; 1991). Seeing the neglect of spirituality in modern psychology's view of human nature, he advocated for a psychology that would synthesize personality study with meditative/spiritual study so that his patients could benefit along both dimensions of growth. He recognized that certain personality patterns can unconsciously harm both self-care and spiritual health and that anyone interested in spirituality needs to also gain greater knowledge of their personality.

This insight brought an attitude that self-awareness increases an individual's ability to make positive choices and changes. Internationally, his insights have been applied by a wide range of professionals in fields as various as diabetes care (Schaub & Simon, 2018), executive coaching (Whitmore, 2002), addictions recovery (Schaub & Schaub, 2013), psychotherapy (Rosselli & Vanni, 2014), and nurse coaching (Schaub & White, 2015). Assagioli's psychosynthesis posits an understanding that consciousness is energy and that cultivating the inner skill to direct consciousness-energy into adaptive mental patterns and away from self-defeating patterns is a health practice. The training of this inner skill is now being recognized in the latest neuroscientific discoveries about different brain regions and the need to strengthen the brain's executive center (Hoezel et al., 2011). In addition, Assagioli's teaching of the objective existence of a transpersonal or higher consciousness in each person and its positive implications for health is now being verified by studies of the "oneness" center of the brain (Newberg & Waldman, 2017). Overall, Assagioli's work provides health professionals with a secular and culturally adaptable approach to engaging with the spiritual potentials in their patients.

Transpersonal Psychology

Transpersonal psychology is a branch of psychology that recognizes and accepts spirituality as an important dimension of the human psyche and of the universal scheme of things (Grof, 1992). Meaning *beyond the personality*, transpersonal refers to the capacity of human nature to go beyond the ordinary mind and ordinary body and to have spiritual, mystical, and energetic experiences that inspire and illuminate people's lives. Historically, religious and spiritual groups have advocated beliefs and methods to awaken these beneficial experiences. European psychiatrists, Carl Jung and Roberto Assagioli, pioneered the use of a transpersonal perspective into their clinical work. They asked how do these experiences happen, what part of the self is involved, what are the neuroscience correlates of such experiences, and how can they safely be stimulated by a health professional.

In the 1970s, pioneering nursing theorists Martha Rogers and her Theory of Unitary Human Beings and Jean Watson and her Theory of Transpersonal Caring and Caring Science (Frisch & Potter, 2016) understood and described how this expanded awareness was vital to health promotion. Reductions in fear even in the face of serious illness, increases the quality of life, increases a sense of life purpose, increases feelings of connection and compassion all indicating that transpersonal experiences are an important contribution to healthcare knowledge. Current neuroscience research, via the recent surge of interest in the medical benefits of meditation, is now investigating meditative states of consciousness and suggesting a "higher" or "oneness" center of the brain that is involved in such transpersonal experiences. In this way, transpersonal psychology represents one intersection of science and spirituality and contributes to the mind–body–spirit perspective of many nursing theories.

Transtheoretical Model Stages of Change

The Transtheoretical Model (TTM) also known at the Stages of Change is a integrative theory to assess the readiness of a person to change. Before the groundbreaking work of Prochaska, Norcross, and DiClemente (1994). a healthcare consumer's readiness was not really discussed in any organized way (Prochaska, Norcross, & DeClemente, 1994). Prochaska, fueled by a personal curiosity about why some people change and others do not, led his team in a study to this phenomenon. The stages of change or the transtheoretical model of change has several key concepts such as stages of change, processes of change, levels of change, and decisional balance.

Coaching has benefited from this model immensely since it has five stages of change matched to five levels of intervention.

1. **Precontemplation**. The first stage includes people who deny they have a problem. They might feel that they don't know how to make a change (internal resistance) or blame someone else for them not being able to build a healthy habit (external resistance) such as a person cannot quit smoking because his wife smokes. Consciousness raising is the strategy to encourage them to move to the next stage and can be given in the form of information.

2. **Contemplation**. The second stage refers to a person who does want to make a change but not right now so the date for the shift might be in about 3 months. Questions about what needs to be ready for the change to occur might be helpful at this stage. Sometimes the person needs to wait for the right circumstances to be in place. For instance, someone might not want to stop smoking during a stressful divorce.

3. **Preparation**. The third stage occurs when the person is ready to make a change. If preparation does not occur, lasting change is less likely to happen. This is the stage of transition that is well suited for coaching.

4. **Action**. The fourth stage is defined as the time when the individual makes the change. Coaching is a fit for this step as well.

5. **Maintenance**. The fifth stage is a period when the person is learning how to truly integrate the change into his or her life. Sometimes the person does the new behavior and other times the individual goes back to the old pattern. This is a risky time for lasting behavior change because one can easily think that they could still do the old behavior. Because of this attitude, they might slip backwards and loose the new behavior. Coaching is well suited to help clients manage this stage so that the transition moves into the new way to be.

The application of their work touches many aspects of healthcare. For instance, before their work was released, eighty percent of the money used to help people change behavior was spent in precontemplation which had twenty percent of the people. This group was not ready to change so this strategy was not effective. Once the nurse coach and client discussed the Stages of Change and where the resistance occurs, health promotion strategies begin to unfold.

Each stage reflects not only a period of time but also a set of tasks that must be completed if the person is to move to the next stage. The journey requires the 5 steps of **Psych** (get ready); **Prep** (plan before leaping); **Perspire** (take action); **Persevere** (mange slips), and **Persist** (maintain change; Norcross, 2012).

Reflective Practice

Reflective practice reviews and evaluates context against which experience is positioned (Johns, 1995). Reflection can be a means of empowerment when practitioners are committed and take responsibility for their own practice. This involves reconstructing and reorienting deeply engrained personally held constructs. Reflection relies on courage to face one's own misperceptions in order to open-up and overcome one's barriers than can be a detriment to skillful practice and an unproductive pattern of relating. Living a vision of competent practice is more than adhering to set minimum standards and goes beyond knowledge or skilled based training.

Reflection enhances the core ingredients of empowerment, personal agency, confidence, and responsibility. Nurse coaches acknowledge and appreciate that personal and professional development needs are also associated with more positively perceived teamwork and performance. Reflective practice can enhance clinical reasoning by maintaining a critical view of current practices. There are many strategies to facilitate deeper levels of self awareness. Immersive simulation experiences such as role play or guided reflection can provide an opportunity to reflect on practice to provide safer, more empathetic and compassionate care.

Resilience

Resilience is a term generally used to describe the ability to persevere through hardships to meet goals. Resilience has been cited as a predictor of well-being and generally refers to one's ability to maintain or regain mental health after experiencing adversity (McCraty & Childers, 2010). Resilient individuals exhibit the ability to "bounce back" from stressful and negative emotional experiences. Nurse coaches emphasize resilience as flexible adaptability in the face of challenge.

Physical resilience is reflected in physical flexibility, endurance, and strength. Mental resilience is reflected in one's attention span, mental flexibility, optimistic worldview, and ability to integrate multiple points of view. Emotional resilience is related to one's ability to self-regulate the expression of one's emotions. Spiritual resilience is related to one's commitment to one's core values, the ability to trust one's intuition, and tolerance of other's values and beliefs (Hess, et al., 2013). While questions remain concerning the development of resilience (Atkinson, Martin, Rankin, 2009; Gillespie, Chaboyer, & Willis, 2007), there are nurse scholars who contend that development of resilience has the potential to improve clinical outcomes (Chaboyer & Wallis, 2007; Warelow, 2005).

The nurse coach helps clients build personal strengths through strategies such as how to build positive and nurturing relationships; maintaining positivity; developing emotional insight; achieving life balance and spirituality; and, becoming more reflecttive. The dimensions of resilience (which include self-efficacy, self-control, ability to engage support and help, learning from difficulties, and persistence despite blocks to progress) are all recognized as qualities that are important for nurse coaches.

Sense-of-Coherence Theory

The Sense-of-Coherence Theory (SOC) is a theory of salutogenesis. Developed by Antonovsky (1996), it represents a perspective that is different from a traditional pathogenic orientation of health. The focus is on what makes a person move toward health. The focus is on the story of the person rather than the diagnosis. The person is understood as an open system in active interaction with the environment (both external and internal conditions) (Langeland et al., 2007, p. 277). A sense of coherence concerns the extent to which one has a feeling of confidence that one's internal and external environments are predictable and can be explained. The sense-of-coherence theory contains three components: comprehensibility, manageability, and meaningfulness.

Comprehensibility refers to the ability to understand situations. Manageability refers to a person's perception that needed resources are available. Meaningfulness refers to the extent to which life is perceived as making sense emotionally and is often considered the most important component (Langeland et al., 2007). A sense of coherence will influence the motivation to engage in self-management of one's health (Chenworth et al., 2008). It is also relevant to the elevated levels of distress and worry that is experienced by many students and young people in general. Davidson et al. (2012) use this salutogenic paradigm to create to create a program for first year college students as a protective element in the demanding academic system they were in. Results demonstrated that the participants experienced higher levels of hope and self-efficacy as a result of the treatment. This is significant in regard to a movement toward the health and well-being of the students.

Self-Efficacy Theory

Self-Efficacy Theory was developed over 20 years of research by the Stanford psychologist, Albert Bandura (1977). The basic belief is that those patients with high self-efficacy expectations can achieve health goals whereas, conversely, those with low self-efficacy expectations will not be incentivized to face challenges, leading to the importance of teaching and training patients in the development of self-efficacy skills and attitudes. The teaching and training of self-efficacy mirrors the coaching approach in that determining goals, making an action plan, predicting likely challenges and imagining strategies to overcome those challenges if they arise (Jordan, 2013). Above all, the self-efficacy model asks for a willingness to practice new behaviors even while uncertain that the goals can be achieved. In this act of willingness, self-efficacy is said to be discovered and utilized.

General self-efficacy refers to one's belief that he or she can handle a broad spectrum of stresses and demands. *Specific* self-efficacy refers to the multiple variables that are at play in taking on a particular challenge or task (Luszczynska et al., 2010). A study examined how self-efficacy impacted dietary behaviors. Improvements in self-efficacy reflected some improvement in behavior changes. While this was not the only factor the study noted that it was a factor when determining which behavioral interventions were most effective (Nothwehr, 2006).

Vulnerability Model

The Vulnerability Model (VM) was first presented by Bonney and Richard Schaub in the middle 1980s to drug and alcohol treatment centers and wrote their first book about it, *Healing Addictions: The Vulnerability Model of Recovery*, in 1997. Vulnerability is a term for the factual human condition of being subject to change and loss at any time, a fact of life that especially reveals itself in times of illness (Schaub, 2016). This theoretical model examines the relation between self-esteem and depression. The health professional is therefore continually encountering people who are in states of active vulnerability. Knowledge of the typical reactions to vulnerability is essential in understanding clients' emotions, attitudes and behaviors toward both professional care and self-care.

The Vulnerability Model defines in depth the three predictable reactions to vulnerability as follows:

- **Willful** (angry and controlling)
- **Will-less** (fearful and escapist)
- **Willing** (realistic and collaborative)

These three predictable reactions provide insight to the varied ways people respond to fears and challenges. Beyond addictions recovery, the Vulnerability Model has since been adapted to trauma recovery, young adult anxiety, cancer care and other clinical issues. Understanding of vulnerability and the reactions it evokes has the potential to illuminate both the professional/patient relationship and the professional's work satisfaction and self-care. Included in this view are health professionals' own reactions to the vulnerability they witness and are exposed to every single day that can lead to compassion fatigue and burnout.

Appendix D
Interventions Frequently Used in Nurse Coaching Practice

Affirmation	Healing Touch	Presence
Appreciative Inquiry	Holistic Self-Assessments	Probing Questions
Aromatherapy	Humor and Laughter	Reflection
Art	Intention	Reiki
Celebration	Journaling	Relaxation Modalities
Client Assessments	Meditation	Rituals of Healing
Cognitive Reframing	Mindfulness Practice	Self-Care Interventions
Contracts	Motivational Interviewing	Self-Reflection
Deep Listening	Movement	Silence
Drawing	Music	Somatic Awareness
Energy Healing	Observation	Sound
Exercise	Play	Stories
Flower Essences	Powerful Questions	Therapeutic Touch
Goal Setting	Prayer	Visioning
Guided Imagery		

© 2021 Mary Elaine Southard, Barbara M. Dossey, Linda Bark & Bonney Gulino Schaub. Used with permission.

Appendix E
American Holistic Nurses Credentialing Corporation (AHNCC) Nurse Coach Certification Process

Initiating Nursing Alliances

In 2012, the authors of *The Art and Science of Nursing Coaching: A Provider's Guide to Scope and Competencies* (Hess et al., 2013), known as the Professional Nurse Coach Workgroup (PNCW), entered into a conversation with the American Holistic Nurse Credentialing Corporation (AHNCC) regarding the paradigm shift toward health and wellness inherent in the Affordable Care Act, and the importance of developing a role and certification program for the professional nurse coach. Given that Holistic Nurses specialize in the practice of health and wellness, it was mutually determined that AHNCC was the appropriate venue for a national certification program for professional nurse coaches. After lengthy discussion, the PNCW entered an agreement with AHNCC whereby AHNCC would sponsor the work of the PNCW in exchange for the rights to establish a national certification process for the nurse coach.

Certification Examination Development

The AHNCC and the Professional Testing Corporation (PTC, n.d.) of New York collaborated to develop a set of competencies, extrapolated from the literature and in accordance with ANA's *Nursing: Scope and Standards of Practice, Second Edition* (ANA, 2010) that now follows the ANA *Nursing: Scope and Standards of Practice, Third Edition* (ANA, 2015) and AHNA and ANA's *Holistic Nursing: Scope and Standards of Practice, Third Edition* (AHNA & ANA, 2018). The competencies, reviewed by expert panels, were revised until approved, and then used to develop a Role-Delineation Study (RDS).

Based on the findings of the RDS, a multiple-step process, overseen by PTC, was used to develop the examination. This rigorous process included: item-writing to assess specified competencies, item-reviews to assess content validity, and an exam-development process to assess content and construct validity. Item-analysis to assess for reliability is undertaken following the administration of each examination. The results from the RDS were used to guide the development of the first Nurse Coach Certification Examination. The

Nurse Coach Examination that was offered in February 2013. Another RDS was conducted in 2016 and the new form of the examination was offered in 2017. The next RDS will be conducted in 2021.

The Nurse Coach Board Certification Examination is based on the *Core Competencies* (reference here) validated in the RDS. These competencies are offered within the context of the AHNA Standards and Core Values. The examination blueprint is formatted based on the weighting of the competencies, which were determined by RDS findings. More detailed information can be found in the *Nurse Coach Certification Examination Handbook and Credentialing and Application* (n.d.). The AHNCC Nurse Coach examination blueprint shows the weighting of the items by Core Values as follows:

Core Value 1. Nurse Coach Philosophy, Theories, and Ethics (25%)

Core Value 2. Nurse Coaching Process (41%)

Core Value 3. Nurse Coach Communication and Coaching Environment (20%)

Core Value 4. Education, Research, and Leadership (8%)

Core Value 5. Self-Reflection, Self-Assessment, and Self-Care (6%)

Additional information is available on the AHNCC website: www.ahncc.org or http://www.ahncc.org/certification/nursecoachnchwnc.html.

Nurse Coach Certification Credentials

The AHNCC recognizes two different Nurse Coach Certifications. Registered nurses that are not AHNCC Holistic Nurse Certified are granted the initials NC-BC (Nurse Coach-Board Certified). Registered nurses that are AHNCC Holistic Nurse Board Certified, and have demonstrated their expertise in health and wellness, are therefore granted the initials HWNC-BC (Health and Wellness Nurse Coaches).

Appendix F
Global Health and Nurse Coaching

Professional nurse coaches are keenly aware that everything that humans do contributes to national and global healthcare transformation or its very destruction. As the world and its economies become increasingly globalized, including extensive international travel and commerce, it is necessary to think about health in a global context. This includes strengthening our understanding of the ethical principles and guideline of global health nursing practice. A recent study identified 10 ethical principles for global health nursing practices and 30 statements for ethical guidelines in global health nursing (McDermott-Levy, Leffers, & Mayaka, 2018). These ten principles addressed beneficence, nonmaleficence, dignity, respect, autonomy, social justice, and professional practice. The 30 guidelines offer more specific actions nurses must consider when working in global settings.

Nurse coaches have made shifts in their consciousness to become role models, health communicators, and health diplomats who are coaching to achieve a healthier humanity—local and global. This calls nurses to recognize that we are one mind, one health, and one planet, and to commit our pledge to planetary citizenship (Rosa, 2017).

This view of global, planetary citizenship is seen as a means to improve relationships, increase environmental awareness, and develop a world based on respect and social justice. Nurses are challenged to engage in diverse areas and provide solutions that create concrete changes in policy, multisector equities for the global population, and the eradication of poverty (Rosa, 2017). This is fundamental if we are to achieve healthy people living on a healthy planet (Nightingale Initiative for Global Health, n.d.).

Professional nurse coaches focus on new models of care delivery that move from a disease management model to a philosophy of wholeness and human flourishing. Their engagement with individual healthcare consumers that includes individual and group coaching can significantly reduce healthcare costs and mortality (Hess, et al., 2013). Nurse coaches are strategically positioned to skillfully partner with healthcare consumers to assess, strategize, plan, and evaluate progress toward negotiated goals for behavioral change, and to promote healthy lifestyles, recognizing that awareness, choice, and intention are essential if healthy lifestyle behaviors are to be sustained (Dossey, Luck, & Schaub, 2015).

Professional nurse coaches are leaders in engaging healthcare consumers in self-care and adoption of healthy life style behaviors that lead to improved healthcare outcomes. The American Nurses Association (ANA) Healthy Nurse Health Nation™ Healthy Nurse Healthy Nation, n.d.) has empowered nurse coaches' awareness of personal self-development and being a role model for increased health awareness and making healthier lifestyle choices. New efforts must be implemented to prevent disease and to create strategies for a healthy and fit world, recognizing that prevention must become part of daily life and to translate the Healthy People 2030 framework, objectives, goals, principles, and strategies for all communities into action as discussed next.

Healthy People 2030

Healthy People 2030 (Healthy People 2030, n.d.) is the fifth 10-year Healthy People decade starting in 1980, to improve the health and well-being of people in the United States. There has been strong collaboration across agencies at the national, state, local, and tribal levels, and with the private and public health sectors. Specific achievements include reducing major causes of death such as heart disease and cancer; reducing infant and maternal mortality; reducing risk factors like tobacco smoking, hypertension, and elevated cholesterol; and increasing childhood vaccinations. All of these endeavors point directly to Nightingale's legacy for today.

Nurse Coaching and Florence Nightingale's Legacy for the 21st Century

Florence Nightingale (1820–1910), the founder of modern secular nursing and the first nurse theorist, began to ponder what nursing could be in the future (Dossey, 2010). She left nurses—as 21st-century Nightingales—with an expansive worldview of how to carry forward her vision of health, including what we recognized today as social and environmental determinants of health. She identified environmental health determinants as clean air, water, food, houses, etc. and social health determinants as poverty, education, family relationships, employment—local to global.

Nightingale saw 19th century problems and created 20th century solutions. Nurses today have seen both 20th and 21st century problems. We can create 21st century solutions by addressing the concerns we find in our own personal lives, and in our families, homes, clinics, hospitals, communities, and in the grassroots-to-global issues.

Nurse coaches are engaged leaders that have increased public concern for global health issues. They strive to inform, engage, and empower nurses, midwives, and concerned citizens to advocacy by translating the United Nations 17 Sustainable Development Goals 2030 Agenda. Nightingale foresaw the complex global problems and challenges and anticipated the 17 UN Sustainable Development Goals (SDGs) (UN, n.d.) as discussed next.

United Nations 17 Sustainable Development Goals 2030 Agenda

As we prepare to globally celebrate the Bicentenary of Florence Nightingale's birth in the year 2020, her insights still have fresh relevance to a new vision for achieving a healthy world community—through "we the peoples of the United Nations"—and the 17 United Nations Sustainable Development Goals (SDGs) 2030 Agenda.

"Health" is the common thread that runs through all 17 UN SDGs. Professional nurse coaches are part of the 29 million nurses and midwives of the world (Haddad & Butler, 2018). They also recognized that these 17 UN SDGs are addressing climate change through a nursing lens (Lilienfeld, Nicholas, Breakey, & Corless, 2018). These goals are directly related to the work of all nurses everywhere, many of whom are engaged in coaching people to find local solutions that can impact health at the global level (Rosa, Upvall, Beck, & Dossey, 2019).

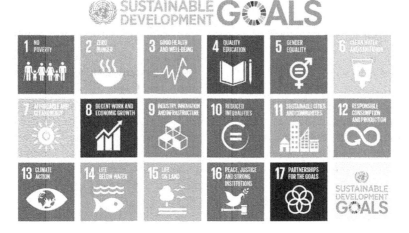

FIGURE 1. United Nations Sustainable Development Goals (SDGs).

The 17 U.N. Sustainable Development Goals Icons used with full attribution and according to UN.org Guidelines (www.un.org/sustainabledevelopment/news/communications-material)

As the largest global health profession, nurses are critical to the health of the nation and the world (WHO, n.d.). The 2018 Gallup Poll declared nurses in the U.S. as the most trusted of all the professions (Gallup, 2020). Nurses are credible sources of health information and are more likely to educate and coach healthcare consumers about improved health and to advocate for the "Global Goals" needed both at home and around the world. In the next section we explore how nurse coaches can work and contribute their knowledge, standards, and competencies to the mission of five global nursing organizations.

Professional Nurses Coaches and Global Nursing Organizations

Nurse coaches are strengthening their commitment to planetary citizenship (Rosa, 2017) and their personal commitment to healthy people living on a healthy planet (Nightingale Declaration, n.d.). Bringing these "Global Goals" back around to each of us as individuals, Nightingale always encouraged her nurses to be as healthy as possible so as to reach their highest potential and explore how they can contribute to a healthy world and also to look toward future with advocacy and meaningful engagement (Beck, Rosa, & Dossey, 2019).

On January 30, 2019, the World Health Organization (WHO) declared that 2020 would be *The Year of the Nurse and Midwife* (Nursing Now, n.d.) to feature their advocacy and service for healthy world and universal healthcare. Currently five major international organizations are collaborating together and in many different partnerships to achieve a healthy world.

Nursing NOW

Nursing Now (Nursing Now, n.d.) is a 3-year Burdett Trust for Nursing global campaign, in collaboration with the International Council of Nurses (ICN) and the World Health Organization (WHO) to raise the voices of nurses worldwide to improve health and well-being. They are empowering nurses and midwives who are at the heart of most health teams to be empowered in their crucial role in health promotion, disease prevention, and treatment. As the health professionals who are closest to the community nurses and midwives have a particular role in developing new models of community-based care and supporting local efforts to promote health and prevent disease.

International Council of Nurses

The International Council of Nurses (ICN) is a federation of more than 130 national nurses associations representing the 20 millions of nurses worldwide (ICN, n.d.). Founded in 1899, ICN is the world's first and widest reaching international organization for health professionals. Operated by nurses, ICN works to ensure the quality of nursing care for all, sound health policies globally, the advancement of nursing knowledge, and the presence worldwide of a respected nursing profession and a competent and satisfied nursing workforce. Professional nurse coaches can contribute to the quality of nursing care, influence healthcare policy, and be involved in scientific advances.

Global Network of WHO Collaborating Centres (WHOCCs) for Nursing and Midwifery Development

To organize nursing and midwifery leadership, the Global Network of WHO Collaborating Centres (WHOCCs) for Nursing and Midwifery Development is an independent, international, non-for-profit, voluntary organization, currently comprising 44 institutions of excellence, from the six regions of the World Health Organization (WHO) (WHOCC, n.d.). Founded in 1988, the Network strives to enhance the collaborative activities of Nursing and Midwifery Collaborating Centers, supporting WHO's efforts towards Health for All (Global Network of WHO Collaborating Centers, n.d.). Professional nurse coaches can include coaching skills in the provision of direct care to mothers and infants as this sits at the core of one of today's most critical global health concerns. Clearly nursing practice has been and must continue to be integrally involved in this challenge.

CGFNS International

The CGFNS International (also known as the Commission on Graduates of Foreign Nursing Schools) is to serve the global community through programs and services that verify and promote the knowledge-based practice competency of healthcare professionals. The Commission on Graduates for Foreign Nursing Schools (CGFNS) began in 1977. The vision of CGFNS is to be the premier source of credentials evaluation and professional development services that provide strategic value and direction to healthcare professionals worldwide (CGFNS, n.d.). The Professional nurse coach recognizes the importance of sound credentialing and deepening the professional development of the nurse.

Sigma Theta Tau International

Sigma Theta Tau International (STTI), founded in 1922 with 135,000 active members, has as its mission to support the learning, knowledge and professional development of nurses committed to making a difference in health worldwide (STTI, n.d.). The STTI vision is to create a global community of nurses who lead in using knowledge, scholarship, service and learning to improve the health of the world's people. The importance of the professional nurse coach role has been recognized by STTI, as evidenced by the organization's publication of *Coaching in Nursing* (Donner & Wheeler, 2009).

Appendix G
An Electronic Health Record (EHR) for Professional Nurse Coaching Practice*

Evidence-based practice of nurse coaching requires the process of collecting, analyzing, and tracking information about patient outcomes, nursing interventions and competencies. Assessment, diagnosis, outcomes identification, planning, implementation, and evaluation are clearly central to the nursing role.

In large healthcare institutions like hospitals and government bureaucracies, these information processes are often managed by complex Electronic Health Record (EHR) systems. Unfortunately, most EHRs are designed for administrators, insurance companies and funders, not the people who are actually providing and receiving services. EHRs are a major source of stress among clinicians (Collier, 2017) and often take large amounts of time that could be spent on serving patients. A recent systematic review found that upon implementation of an EHR system, nurses documentation increased from 9% to 23% of their time (Baumann, Baker, & Elshaug, 2018).

The design challenge of EHRs is even more difficult for holistic and integrative nursing, which does not fit reductive, rigid approaches to patient management. The utilization of an EHR that captures the client story and the practice of a nurse coach needs to be tailored and flexible.

So what are the options for nurse coaches? There is broad consensus that paper records are inadequate for improving patient care, promoting safe practice, and enabling communication between patients and multiple providers (Palabindala, Pamarthy, & Jonnalagadda, 2016), and it is not enough just to convert from paper records to digital records. Unstructured clinical notes in a database or Word documents are almost as bad as paper records for the purpose of tracking patient progress and improving service quality.

Professional nurse coaches' practice requires some form of structured note-taking, not only for clinical assessment (establishing relationship and identifying readiness to change), planning (individual goals), and implementation but also for continual evaluation (outcomes) and quality improvement (self-reflection).

---

* ©2021 David Gotlib & Mary Elaine Southard. Used with permission.

Creating a Usable EHR for Nurse Coaching

KoNote is an open source EHR that was designed around the needs of clinicians and their patients. It was developed over several years by David Gotlib, a practicing psychiatrist, with a software development team and is in use in several health settings. The software is supported by a Canadian nonprofit (LogicalOutcomes, www.logicaloutcomes.com).

In 2018, Gotlib and Gillian Kerr, a clinical psychologist and President of Logical Outcomes, worked with a group of doctoral nursing students associated with the University of Minnesota to customize it for nursing practice. A further customization was created specifically for nurse coaching, led by Mary Elaine Southard.

The customization has been designed to support nurse coaches through assessment, diagnosis, outcomes identification, health promotion, and evaluation in a way that reflects a holistic, patient-centered perspective.

KoNote in general is based on several design principles:

- EHRs should be designed for the needs of the patients and service providers. Other users (like payers) are secondary.

- EHRs should help service providers to improve their practice.

- EHRs should minimize data entry burden as much as possible while providing useful information that can be tracked over time.

- Each metric should either be an effective intervention in itself (such as specific evidence-based indicators on daily nutritional goals) or lead to better services (such as patient satisfaction with the session).

- Service providers should be able to create relevant metrics within a clinical plan without hiring an external information technology expert. For example, a nurse coach may want to track a patient's social contacts with friends, or their spending habits.

- Data should be interoperable with other systems to avoid vendor lock-in.

- EHRs must protect the privacy and security of sensitive personal information.

The nurse coaching template builds on the KoNote base by creating a basic structure for note-taking that can be quickly revised by each nurse coach to match their own practice. Here is a screenshot of a progress note:

KoNote
Progress Note

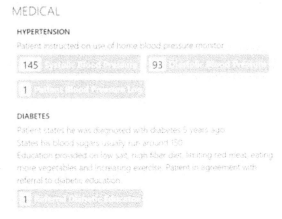

MEDICAL

HYPERTENSION

Patient instructed on use of home blood pressure monitor

145   93

1

DIABETES

Patient states he was diagnosed with diabetes 5 years ago.
States his blood sugars usually run around 150.
Education provided on low salt, high fiber diet, limiting red meat, eating
more vegetables and increasing exercise. Patient in agreement with
referral to diabetic education.

1

The initial interview screen looks simple enough; just a list of open text questions. After the initial interview, these questions can be deactivated. Future progress notes will ask about key metrics that can be tracked in each section.

Viewing Meaningful Data in an EHR

KoNote visualizes the metrics automatically, so that the nurse coach can track meaningful change over time. The following examples:

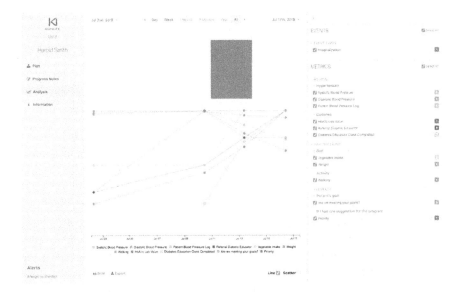

And another view:

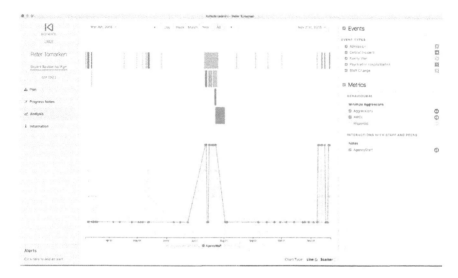

The process of nurse coaching is collaborative and sharing a visual depiction of the individuals self-determined goals and trajectory can augment the knowledge, behavior, or status of the goal. Longitudinal trends can be shown to correlate with resistance and open up dialogue for deeper understanding and discovery.

A well-designed EHR can be a joy rather than a burden to use. One of the first adopters was the Griffin Centre in Toronto, a nonprofit mental health agency providing services to youth and adults. Deanna Dannell, Chief Operating Officer, states:

"In the short time that we have implemented KoNote in our treatment program we have seen the benefits of this tool from both the staff and client level. Staff using this tool have reported improved documentation that has enhanced our ability to collect data and evaluate client goals and treatment. It has supported a consistent and shared vision of client treatment within the team and the consultants who support the direct service delivery. It has allowed for consultants to have access to accurate data in a timely manner, which results in improved consultation with team members and the creation of responsive interventions."

Clients and family also benefit from KoNote. Allowing clients and families to visually see their progress and the events that contribute to their success will enhance the engagement of clients and families in their treatment. Clients and families become active participants in their treatment which increase their ability to sustain their improvements once leaving our services.

"KoNote has filled a void in our organization. It has created a nimble electronic client record that can easily meet the unique needs of our intensive treatment programs. It has been an easy to learn/easy to use tool for our front line workers. Management staff have reported improved confidence and comfort in their oversight of the treatment program."

Appendix H
Groundwork for Emerging Competencies for Graduate and Advanced Practice Nurse Coach: Setting the Stage*

This *draft* of emerging competencies, based on structure, quality and certification of entry level nurse coaching expands the breath and depth of how advanced practice nurses encompass the skills of advanced practice with additional coaching skills. The scope statements below are intended to encourage research and delineate further confirmation of the benefits of advanced practice nurses when coaching complex patient situations and goals.

This document can serve as a framework for opportunities and action items to fully articulate and validate the return on investment of nurse coaching from an advanced practice role. Embedded are advanced coaching skills that will require the rigor of certification in the near future.

Six Step Nurse Coaching Process

Step 1: Assessment
Additional competencies for the graduate level-prepared nurse coach

In addition to the competencies for the basic-level nurse coach, the graduate-prepared nurse coach:

- ▶ Obtains and accurately documents a relevant holistic health history based on client narrative to assess all aspects of the patient's health status, including health promotion, health protection and disease prevention;

- ▶ Performs a comprehensive physical, mental and spiritual assessment;

---

* ©2021 Mary Elaine Southard, Barbara M. Dossey, Linda Bark & Bonney Gulino Schaub. Used with permission.

- Explores the narrative meanings of symbolic language expressed in sensations, images, dreams, rituals and prayers as part of the health consumer experience; and

- Employs aggregate-level data and current research, thinking, and theory to articulate health challenges and issues.

Additional competencies for the advanced practice prepared nurse coach

In addition to the above competencies for the graduate-level nurse coach, the advanced practice nurse coach:

- Uses advanced nurse coaching assessments, knowledge, and skills to facilitate desired change, improve, maintain, and sustain health conditions for health consumer's growth and self-development;

- Analyzes the relationship between normal physiology and specific system alterations using pattern recognition, intuition, and other ways of knowing;

- Identifies and analyzes factors that may be barriers to health; i.e., genetics, family, environment, trauma, psychodynamics, culture and ethnicity, spiritual beliefs and practices, physiological processes, coping skills, cognition, developmental stage, socioeconomic status, gender, or substance abuse;

- Collects data from multiple sources using holistic assessment techniques that are appropriate to the patient's language, culture, and developmental stage, including, but not limited to, energetic assessments, standardized instruments, or genograms;

- Assesses the impact of stressors as barriers to change, as patient identifies physiological, emotional, or spiritual manifestations to health;

- Synthesizes, prioritizes, and documents relevant data in a retrievable form;

- Ensures patient safety through appropriate referral, collaboration, and interface with additional provider per permission of patient; and

- Applies therapeutic communication strategies based on theories and research evidence to reduce emotional distress, facilitate cognitive and behavioral change, and foster personal growth.

Step 2: Diagnosis
Additional competencies for the graduate level-prepared nurse coach

In addition to the competencies for the basic-level nurse coach, the graduate-prepared nurse coach:

▶ Assists staff to include client narratives to recognize patterns in the diagnostic process;

▶ Models and role models coaching therapeutic relationship to promote positive clinical outcomes; and

▶ Monitors own emotional reaction and behavioral responses of coaching sessions through self-awareness, reflective journaling, and 360 degree evaluation (Comack et al., 2018).

Additional competencies for the advanced practice nurse coach

In addition to the above competencies for the graduate-level nurse coach, the advanced practice nurse coach:

▶ Interprets and individualizes therapies to promote knowledge, understanding, and effective management of health problems and disorders;

▶ Employs aggregate-level data to articulate health challenges and issues of healthcare and organizational systems; and

▶ Monitors complex data and information obtained during coaching session to assist with health consumer's desired behavioral changes.

Step 3: Outcome Identification
Additional competencies for the graduate level-prepared nurse coach

In addition to the competencies for the basic-level nurse coach, the graduate-prepared nurse coach:

▶ Incorporates healthcare consumer satisfaction, the person's understanding and meaning in her/his unique patterns and process, quality of life, cost, practice, effectiveness, and values; and

▶ Integrates scientific evidence and nurse coach best practices to achieve expected outcomes.

Additional competencies for the advanced practice nurse coach

In addition to the above competencies for the graduate-level, the advanced practice nurse coach:

- ▶ Develops a treatment plan, together with the patient, based on bio-psychosocial theories, evidence-based standards of care, and practice guidelines;

- ▶ Identifies, measures, and monitors clinical related behavioral outcomes to determine the effectiveness of coaching interventions; and

- ▶ Evaluates the impact of coaching interventions to determine own novice-to-expert coaching model.

Step 4: Planning
Additional competencies for the graduate level-prepared nurse coach

In addition to the competencies for the basic-level nurse coach, the graduate-prepared nurse coach:

- ▶ Identifies nurse coach assessment strategies, therapeutic interventions, therapeutic effects, and side effects that reflect current nurse coach research;

- ▶ Uses narrative and symbolic language, including, but not limited to, storytelling, journals, word associations, dreams, and rituals to explore the individuals choices, possibilities, and options;

- ▶ Designs, in partnership with the healthcare consumer, strategies to address complex needs in order to minimize the development of complications; and

- ▶ Engages in and collaborates with others in the conduct of nurse coaching research to discover, examine and test knowledge, theories and evidence-based approaches to nurse coaching practice.

Additional competencies for the advanced practice nurse coach

In addition to the competencies for the graduate level-prepared nurse coach, the advanced practice nurse coach:

▶ Integrates nurse coaching assessment strategies, diagnostic strategies, and therapeutic interventions reflecting current evidence-based knowledge and practice; and

▶ Provides consultation to healthcare providers and other colleagues to enhance quality and cost effective services to effect change in organizational systems.

Step 5: Implementation

Additional competencies for the graduate-level prepared nurse coach

In addition to the competencies for the basic-level nurse coach, the graduate-prepared nurse coach:

▶ Supports collaboration with nursing colleagues and other disciplines to implement nurse coaching strategies to cocreate plans for individuals, families, groups, and communities that integrate biomedical and integrative approaches for health and well-being;

▶ Uses nurse coaching principles and engages in traditional and complementary/integrative evidence-based treatments, therapies, procedures, and approaches that are compatible with the healthcare consumer's beliefs, values, choices, cultural preferences, and norms;

▶ Applies quality nurse coaching principles while articulating methods, tools, performance measures, and standards as they relate to implementation of the plan;

▶ Translates nurse coaching evidence into practice; and

▶ Uses nurse coaching theory-driven approaches and other interprofessional-related coaching theories for effective organizational or system changes.

Additional competencies for the advanced practice nurse coach

In addition to the above graduate level-prepared nurse coach competencies, the advanced practice nurse coach:

▶ Provides clinical consultation for healthcare consumers and professionals utilizing nurse coaching approaches with complex clinical cases to improve care and healthcare consumer.

5A. Coordination of Care
Additional competencies for the graduate level-prepared nurse coach

In addition to the competencies for the basic-level nurse coach, the graduate-prepared nurse coach:

▶ Provides nurse coach information and research for identified panels and populations.

5B. Coordination of Care
Additional competencies for the advanced practice nurse coach

In addition to the competencies for the graduate-level nurse coach, the advanced practice nurse coach:

▶ Synthesizes empirical evidence on risk behaviors, nursing theories, learning theories, change theories, for evidence-based practice, and epidemiology, when designing nurse coaching education information and programs; and

▶ Synthesizes nurse coach data and information to provide system and community support measures to assist with coordination of care.

Step 6: Evaluation
Additional competencies for the graduate level-prepared nurse coach

In addition to the competencies for the basic-level nurse coach, the graduate-prepared nurse coach:

▶ Engages in systematic evaluation process to revise the cocreated plan of care to enhance its effectiveness over time; and

▶ Uses results of the evaluation to make or recommend process policy, procedure, or protocol revisions to improve the cocreated plan of care when needed.

Additional competencies for the advanced practice nurse coach

In addition to the competencies for the graduate-level nurse coach, the advanced nurse coach:

▶ Identifies, measures, and monitors outcomes and trends to determine the effectiveness of coaching interventions using advanced methods and tools;

▶ Synthesizes evaluation data from the healthcare consumer, community, population, and/or institution to determine the effectiveness of the plan; and

▶ Evaluates, in partnership with the healthcare consumer, the accuracy of the biomedical and nursing diagnoses, and the effectiveness of the intervention in relationship to the healthcare consumer's attainment of evolving outcomes.

Competencies Associated with ANA Standards of Professional Performance

Standard 7: Ethics
Additional competencies for the graduate level-prepared nurse coach

In addition to the competencies for the basic-level nurse coach, the graduate level-prepared nurse coach:

▶ Advocates for the patient's and family's rights regarding involuntary treatment and other medico-legal issues;

▶ Participates with interprofessional teams to evaluate the ethics of risks, benefits, and outcomes of healthcare regimens; and

▶ Actively engage in creating an ecosystem that supports well-being for all life.

Additional competencies for the advanced practice nurse coach

In addition to the competencies for the graduate-level nurse coach, the advanced practice nurse coach:

▶ Analyzes the impact of duty to report to facilitate safe, therapeutic relationships; and

▶ Provides information on the risks, benefits, and outcomes of health-care regimens to allow informed decision-making by the healthcare consumer, including informed consent and informed refusal.

Standard 8: Culturally Congruent Practice
Additional competencies for the graduate level-prepared nurse coach

In addition to the competencies for the basic-level nurse coach, the graduate-prepared nurse coach:

▶ Evaluates nurse coaching and health and wellness tools, instruments, and services provided to culturally diverse populations as to their appropriateness;

▶ Uses nurse coaching and health and wellness tools to identify and act on the cultural and language needs of the healthcare consumer; and

▶ Uses nurse coaching strategies for recruitment and retention to achieve a multicultural workforce.

Additional competencies for the advanced practice nurse coach

In addition to the competencies for the graduate-level nurse coach, the advanced practice nurse coach:

▶ Uses nurse coaching principle and strategies for shared decision-making solutions in planning, prescribing, and evaluating process when the healthcare consumer's cultural preferences and norms may create incompatibility with evidence-based practice and the values, beliefs, and norms of the biomedical culture;

- Engages healthcare consumers, key stakeholders, and others in designing and promoting internal and external cross-cultural partnerships; and

- Conducts nurse coach research that seeks to inquire about the ways in which the biomedical culture can improve consideration of collaboration of the cultural context of healthcare.

Standard 9: Communication
Additional competencies for the graduate level-prepared nurse coach

In addition to the competencies for the basic-level nurse coach, the graduate level-prepared nurse coach:

- Models nurse coach principles and strategies in creating a healthy workforce environment that facilitates and supports effective communication and healing; and

- Articulates and frames communication using meta-view and metaphor to acknowledge strength in the client's foundation.

Additional competencies for the advanced practice nurse coach

In addition to the competencies for the graduate-level nurse coach, the advanced practice nurse coach:

- Advances interprofessional plan-of-care documentation and communication, provides rationales for plan-of-care changes, and collaborative discussions to improve healthcare consumer healthcare outcomes; and

- Participates in interprofessional activities, including, but not limited to, education consultation, management, technological developments, or research, to enhance health and wellness outcomes.

Standard 10: Collaboration
Additional competencies for the graduate level-prepared nurse coach

In addition to the competencies for the basic-level nurse coach, the graduate-prepared nurse coach:

▶ Assists in improving and sustaining collaborative relationships to achieve safe, quality, holistic, whole person-centered care; and

▶ Utilizes nurse coaching principles and strategies to partner with other disciplines to enhance healthcare consumer's health and well-being and outcomes through interprofessional activities such as education, consultation, management, technological development, or research opportunities.

Additional competencies for the advanced practice nurse coach

In addition to the competencies for the graduate level-prepared nurse coach, the advanced practice nurse coach:

▶ Advances the interprofessional plan-of-care communication, rationales for plan-of-care changes and collaborative discussions; and

▶ Manages emergencies, by determining the level of risk, and initiating and coordinating effective emergency care.

Standard 11: Leadership
Additional competencies for the graduate level-prepared nurse coach

In addition to the competencies for the basic-level nurse coach, the graduate-prepared nurse coach:

▶ Demonstrates nurse coaching leadership skills that emphasize ethical and critical decision-making effective working relationships, and a system perspective;

▶ Models expertise in holistic and integrative nurse coaching practice to interprofessional team members and healthcare consumers; and

- Mentors colleagues in the acquisition of nursing coaching knowledge, skills, abilities, and judgment.

Additional competencies for the advanced practice nurse coach

In addition to the competencies for the graduate-level nurse coach, the advanced practice nurse coach:

- Articulates nurse coach principles in a historical, philosophical and scientific context while projecting futures trends for health and wellness coaching leading to healthy people living on a healthy planet; and
- Influences decision-making bodies to improve holistic integrative care, the professional practice environment, and holistic integrative healthcare consumer outcomes.

Standard 12: Education
Additional competencies for the graduate level-prepared nurse coach

In addition to the competencies for the basic-level nurse coach, the graduate-prepared nurse coach:

- Creates nurse coaching curricula and educational programs that teach and clinically supervise students and practicing nurses the foundations of nurse coaching, a step building education theory;
- Evaluates health and wellness coaching information resources including the internet for applicability, accuracy, readability, and comprehensibility to assist healthcare consumer access quality health information; and
- Educates and disseminates nurse coaching research findings to practitioners and the public.

Additional competencies for the advanced practice nurse coach

In addition to the competencies for the graduate-level nurse coach, the advanced practice nurse coach:

▶ Uses current healthcare research findings and other sources of evidence to expand nurse coaching knowledge, competencies, and judgment; to expand nurse coaching performance; to increase knowledge of nurse coaching professional issues and change national standards for practice and trends in integrative care; and

▶ Contributes to the writing for professional practice dissemination of best practice to inform policy, institutions, and state boards of nursing.

Standard 13: Evidence-Based Practice and Research
Additional competencies for the graduate level-prepared nurse coach

In addition to the competencies for the basic-level nurse coach, the graduate-prepared nurse coach:

▶ Creates ways to study the integration of body–mind–spirit–cultural– environment domains to achieve optimal health outcomes; and

▶ Participates in creating clinical practice guidelines related to nurse coaching.

Additional competencies for the advanced practice nurse coach

In addition to the competencies for the graduate-level nurse coach, the advanced practice nurse coach:

▶ Promotes a climate of research and clinical inquiry;

▶ Disseminates research finding through activities such as presenta- tions, publications, consultations, and journal clubs for a variety of audiences to improve holistic integrative care and further develop the foundation and practice of nurse coaching; and

▶ Contributes to nurse coaching knowledge by synthesizing research that discovers, examines, and evaluates current practice, knowledge, theories, philosophies, context, criteria, and creative approaches to improve health consumer and healthcare outcomes.

Standard 14: Quality of Practice
Additional competencies for the graduate level-prepared nurse coach

In addition to the competencies for the basic-level nurse coach, the graduate-prepared nurse coach:

▶ Incorporates nurse coach information in the development, implementation, evaluation, and/or revision of policies, procedures, and guidelines to improve holistic integrative healthcare quality;

▶ Uses nurse coaching data and information in system-level decision-making; and

▶ Evaluates the impact of coaching interventions to determine own novice-to-expert coaching model.

Additional competencies for the advanced practice nurse coach

In addition to the competencies for the graduate-level nurse coach, the advanced practice nurse coach:

▶ Analyzes trends in health and wellness coaching to enhance healthcare quality data, including examination of cultural biases and factors influencing or impacting quality care; and

▶ Uses available health and wellness coaching benchmarks as a means of evaluating nurse coaching practice at all levels of healthcare (individual, departmental, organizational, and community level).

Standard 15: Professional Practice Evaluation
Additional competencies for the graduate level-prepared nurse coach

In addition to the competencies for the basic-level nurse coach, the graduate-prepared nurse coach:

▶ Applies knowledge obtained from advanced coaching preparation, national and global trends, professional organizations, current coaching research, and evidence-based information to evaluate own nurse coaching practice;

▶ Participates in professional and community organizations that influence the holistic health of patients and supports the role of nurse coach; and

▶ Advocates for the role of nurse coach with other healthcare providers, community, state, and federal agencies and the public.

Additional competencies for the advanced practice nurse coach

In addition to the competencies for the graduate-level nurse coach, the advanced practice nurse coach:

▶ Designs quality improvement programs, studies, and research initiatives, to improve nurse coach outcomes in diverse settings; and

▶ Coordinates referral and ongoing access to primary and other health services for healthcare consumers.

Standard 16: Resource Utilization
Additional competencies for the graduate level-prepared nurse coach

In addition to the competencies for the basic-level nurse coach, the graduate level-prepared nurse coach:

▶ Engages organizational and community resources to design and implement health coach interprofessional plans; and

▶ Evaluates health and wellness coaching information resources including the internet for applicability, accuracy, readability, and comprehensibility to assist healthcare consumer access quality health information.

Additional competencies for the advanced practice nurse coach

In addition to the competencies for the graduate level-prepared nurse coach, the advanced practice nurse coach:

▶ Designs innovative nurse coach solutions to use resources effectively and maintain quality; and

▶ Uses evaluation strategies that address cost effectiveness, cost benefit, and efficiency factors associated with nurse coaching practice.

Standard 17: Environmental Health
Additional competencies for the graduate level-prepared nurse coach

In addition to the competencies for the basic-level nurse coach, the graduate-prepared nurse coach:

▶ Creates partnerships that promote sustainable global policies that focus on the prevention of environmental hazards to healthcare consumers and the environment; and

▶ Serves as a content expert related to the environmental health issues on health consumers and communities.

Additional competencies for the advanced practice nurse coach

In addition to the competencies for the graduate-level nurse coach, the advanced practice nurse coach:

▶ Analyzes the impact of social, political, and economic influences on the environment and human health exposures; and

▶ Contributes to conducting research and applying research findings that link environmental hazards and human response patterns.

Appendix I
Extant Nurse Coach and Nurse Coaching Literature Review (1988–2019)

Adams, S. M., Rice, M. J., Jones, S. L., Herzog, E., Mackenxie, L. J., & Olek, L. G. (2018). TeleMental health: Standards, reimbursement, and interstate practice. *Journal of the American Psychiatric Nurses Association, 4*(24), 295–304.	TeleMental Health (TMH) is gaining widespread acceptance in the United States. This article summarizes current evidence regarding TMH risks and benefits, standards of care, practice guidelines, reimbursement, and interstate practice issues pertinent to psychiatric nurses and consumers. DESIGN: A targeted review of literature, current practice, and TMH websites was generated using the following key search words: clinical outcomes, practice guidelines, regulations, interstate practice, and reimbursement.

© 2021 Mary Elaine Southard, Barbara M. Dossey, Linda Bark & Bonney Gulino Schaub. Used with permission. Adapted from Dossey, B. M. & Hess, D. R. (2013). Professional nurse coaching: Advances in national and global transformation. *Global Advances in Health and Medicine, 2*(4), 10–16.

Appendix I

Ahmann, E. (2017). Interventions for ADHD in children and teens: A focus on ADHD coaching. *Pediatric Nursing, 43*(3), 121–131.	This article introduces ADHD coaching as a behavioral intervention with a growing evidence base. A literature search identified 22 studies addressing ADHD coaching, of which 19 examined outcomes; seven of these studies were specific to children and teens. The studies of coaching for young people with ADHD, like those among older individuals, suggest that ADHD coaching is a promising behavioral intervention and a useful component of multimodal treatment. Pediatric nurses can help families understand ADHD; encourage them to engage behavioral intervention(s), including ADHD coaching.
Allison, M. J., & Keller, C. (2004). Self-efficacy intervention effect on physical activity in older adults. *Western Journal of Nursing Research, 26*(1), 31–46.	Nurse coaches used verbal persuasion, monitored achievements, and awareness of physiological arousal to help increase physical activity self-efficacy of older adults (n = 83). It appears that participants received telephone coaching every 2 weeks for 12 weeks.
Ammentorp, J., & Kofoed, P. E. (2010). Coach training can improve the self-efficacy of neonatal nurses: A pilot study. *Patient Education and Counseling, 79*(2), 258–61.	Neonatal nurses were offered a 3-day coaching training to assess their ability to meet the needs of mothers and fathers. Coach training improved nurses' self-efficacy scores by 14.8% in relation to meeting the needs of mothers and fathers.

Bark, L., & Conrad, S. (2015). Nurse coaching is not what I do: It informs who I am. *Beginnings, 35*(4), 1820.	This article explores how coach training can be a transformational experience for the student coach. They ask what happens in nurse coach training that impacts so much of the student's inner and outer worlds. They also address the paradigm shift that many students experience after integrating the principles of coaching into their practice and daily lives.
Beck, D. M., & Dossey, B. M. (2019). In Nightingale's footsteps—Individual to global: From nurse coaches to environmental and civil society activist. *Creative Nursing: A Journal of Values, Issues, Experience, and Collaboration, 25*(3), 1–6.	Florence Nightingale (1820–1910), the famous "lady with the lamp," is indeed the world's most well-known nurse. In our times, now for nearly six decades, the same environmental and social issues that were of concern to Nightingale are understood as key factors in achieving global development and global health. In Nightingale's footsteps, nurse coach leaders and all nurses are 21st century Nightingales that are coaching, informing, and educating for healthy people to be living on a healthy planet.
Beliveau, L. (2004). Comfort coaching. *Canadian Association Nephrology Nurses and Technologists Journal, 14*(2), 35–36.	Coaching was used to encourage, counsel, educate, and support patients. This is a self-reflective narrative of the (nurse) author's experience serving as coach to two women receiving dialysis while also dealing with cancer.

Appendix I

Berg, J., Tichacek, M. J., & Theodorakis, R. (2004). Evaluation of an educational program for adolescents with asthma. *The Journal of School Nursing, 20*(1), 29–35.	Three weeks of individual nurse coaching took place after participating in a Power Breathing program, a 3-week educational program about asthma. Each student met with a nurse coach three times each week for 15 min to help tailor the education program to his/her needs. Coaching was seen as a separate intervention from the educational program.
Berger-Höger, B., Liethmann, K., Mühlhauserm, I., Haastert, B., & Streckelberg, A. (2019). Nurse-led coaching of shared decision-making for women with ductal carcinoma in situ in breast centers: a cluster randomized controlled trial. *International Journal of Nursing Students, 93*, 141–152. doi:10.1016/j.ijnurstu.2019.01.013.	This article investigated whether an informed shared decision-making intervention for women with "ductal carcinoma in situ" comprising an evidence-based decision aid with nurse-led decision coaching enhances the extent of the mutual shared decision-making behavior of patients and professionals regarding treatment options, and to analyze implementation barriers. Fourteen breast centers were randomized to intervention or standard care and 64 patients (partially blinded) were recruited. Nurse-led decision coaching grounded on evidence-based patient information enhances informed shared decision-making.
Bennett, J. A., Perrin, N. A., Hanson, G., Bennett, D., Gaynor, W., Flaherty-Robb, M., Joseph, C., Butterworth, S., & Potempa, K. (2005). Healthy aging demonstration project: Nurse coaching for behavior change in older adults. *Research in Nursing & Health, 28*(3), 187–197.	Two registered nurses provided coaching after receiving 24 h of motivational interviewing training that consisted of didactic instruction and role-playing. Motivational interviewing consisted of: a) expressing empathy; b) supporting self-efficacy; c) working with resistance; and d) acknowledging and working with discrepancy between behavior and goals.

Blackstone, E., Lipson, A. R., & Douglas, S. L. (2019). Closer: A videoconference intervention for distance caregivers of cancer patients. *Research in Nursing and Health*, May 22. doi: 10.1002/nur.21952.	This is an ongoing randomized controlled trial in 32 outpatient ambulatory clinics at a large, urban, comprehensive cancer center. To date, 332 patient-DCG dyads have been enrolled. DCGs must have internet access and have been identified by the patient as a source of support. The intervention period is 4 months. Primary outcome variables are DCG distress, anxiety, depression, burden, self-efficacy, and emotional support. These data are collected electronically at baseline, 4 months, and 6 months. Patient distress, anxiety, and depression are also assessed at these same intervals using brief in-person interviews.

The change in each of the DCG outcomes over time will be examined by a repeated measures analysis of covariance. |
| Booth, J. (2019). Re-imaging the end of life: Self-development & reflective practices for nurse coaches. Falls Church, VA: Living Well Nurse Coaching. | This handbook provides profound reflections and inspirations for nurse coaches. It examines how to navigate serious health illness and death within our complex healthcare system. It provides healing possibilities of reimaging the end of life as a vital, purposeful stage of human development. Many practices of healing such as forgiveness, gratitude, and letting go illustrate how these can become essential parts of care plans. |

Appendix I

Brinkert, R. (2011). Conflict coaching training for nurse managers: A case study of a two-hospital health system. *Journal of Nursing Management, 19*(1), 80–91.	Twenty nurse managers were trained over an 8-month period as conflict coaches and each coached a supervisee. Conflict coaching was a practical and effective means of developing conflict communication competencies of nurse managers and supervisees. This type program works best when support by a positive conflict culture and integrated with other conflict intervention processes.
Butterworth, S., Linden, A., & McClay, W. (2007). Health coaching as an intervention in health management programs. *Disease Management & Health Outcomes, 15*(5), 299–307.	Article provides evidence-based support for the potential role of nurse coaches in tobacco cessation programs. Motivational interviewing methods were used as part of the coaching technique. Coaching was identified as cost effective strategy compared to counseling.
Carrieri-Kohlman, V., Gormley, J. M., Douglas, M. K., Paul, S. M., & Stulbarg, M. S. (1996). Exercise training decreases dyspnea and the distress and anxiety associated with it: Monitoring alone may be as effective as coaching. *CHEST, 110*(6), 1526–1535.	A master's prepared nurse coach provided the coaching. At the beginning of each coaching session, the nurse coach helped participants (n = 51) set goals related to their clinical status. Coaching was based on guided mastery techniques that included vicarious experiences, verbal persuasion, and physiological feedback.
Carrieri-Kohlman, V., Gormley, J. M., Douglas, M. K., Paul, S. M., & Stulbarg, M. S. (2001). Dyspnea and the affective response during exercise training in obstructive pulmonary disease. *Nursing Research, 50*(3), 136–146.	A master's prepared nurse coach provided the coaching. At the beginning of each coaching session, the nurse coach helped participants (n = 45) set goals related to their clinical status. Coaching was based on guided mastery techniques that included vicarious experiences, verbal persuasion, and physiological feedback.

DeCampli, P., Kirby, K. K., & Baldwin, C. (2010). Beyond the classroom to coaching: Preparing new nurse managers. *Critical Care Nursing Quarterly*, *33*(2), 132–137.	A suburban Philadelphia Magnet-designated hospital engaged an experience nurse executive to coach new nurse managers for four months on site. Face-to-face coaching was agreed as the most important component of the program. Having a seasoned coach also helped increase confidence in the new role.
Delaney, C., & Bark, L. (2019). The experience of holistic nurse coaching for patients with chronic conditions. *Journal of Holistic Nursing*. https://journals.sagepub.com/doi/full/10.1177/08980 10119837109#article ShareContainer.	The purpose of this study was to explore and describe the lived experience of adults with chronic conditions receiving holistic nurse coaching. A qualitative phenomenological research design was used for this study. A purposive sample of 15 patients with varied chronic conditions participated. The patients' stories of their experiences with holistic nurse coaching were analyzed using Colaizzi's method of phenomenological analysis. Eight theme clusters emerged when the formulated meanings were organized into the following categories: (1) Seeking Guidance to Navigate Life's Challenges, (2) Entering a Safe Sacred Place, (3) Feeling Empowered and Accountable, (4) Developing Strategies to Access Different Ways of Knowing, (5) Finding the Answers Within, (6) Making Healthy Behavioral Changes, (7) Forming a New Caring Relationship with Self, and (8) Transforming to a Brand-New Approach to Life.
Donner, G., & Wheeler, M. M. (2009). Coaching in nursing: An introduction. Geneva, Switzerland: International Council of Nursing and Indianapolis, IN: The Honor Society of Nursing, Sigma Theta Tau International.	This document provides an overview of professional nurse coaching. This document is based upon the International Coach Federation (ICF) core competencies.

Appendix I

Dossey, B. M., & Luck, S. (2015). Nurse coaching through a nursing lens: The theory of integrative nurse coaching. *Beginnings, 35*(4), 10–13, 25.	The Theory of Integrative Nurse Coaching© (TINC) presents the art and science of integrative nurse coaching. The TINC is a middle-range nursing theory that is best suited to the interactive-integrative paradigm of nursing theories. It is focused in scope on the specific nursing phenomenon of integrative nurse coaching. The TINC includes a designated and validated Integrative Health and Wellness Assessment™.
Dossey, B. M., Luck, S., Schaub, B. G., & Hess, D. R. (2013). Nurse coaching. In B.M. Dossey & L. Keegan, *Holistic nursing: A handbook for practice* (6th ed.) (pp. 189–204). Burlington, MA: Jones & Bartlett Learning.	The evolution of health coaching and nurse coaching introduces the topic of nurse coaching. The professional nurse coach scope of practice and competencies is described, including nurse coaching core values. Application of the Theory of Integral Nursing and the Integrative Nurse Coach Method and Process is applied to a discussion of nurse coaching and change. The nurse coaching process is compared to the nursing process.
Dossey, B. M., & Hess, D. R. (2013). Professional nurse coaching: Advances in national and global transformation. *Global Advances in Health and Medicine, 2*(4), 10–16.	The goals of this review were as follows: 1) to identify how the health and wellness coach role was embedded in nursing practice; 2) to identify areas where nurse coaching skills were used and integrated; 3) to determine how nurse coaches defined their roles, practices, and competencies; 4) to explore emerging trends within professional nurse coaching practice; and 5) to identify areas of future research in nurse coaching.

Dossey, B. M., Luck, S., & Schaub, B. G. (2015). Nurse coaching: Integrative approaches for health and wellbeing. North Miami, FL: International Nurse Coach Association.	This is the first comprehensive nurse coaching textbook that informs practice, education, research, and health policy. Using a nursing lens for health and wellness coaching, this book is an essential guide for nurse coaching. It is organized by the recognized five core values and has 22 chapters and an in-depth Appendices with over 40 lifestyle and health coaching tools and practices.
Dowd, T., Kolcaba, K., & Steiner, R. (2003). The addition of coaching to cognitive strategies: Interventions for persons with compromised urinary bladder syndrome. *Journal of Would, Ostomy, & Continence Nursing, 30*(2), 90–99.	Coaching was used to provide support to patients. Participants (n = 35) received weekly coaching calls for 12 weeks. Coaching enhanced selected outcomes. Information regarding the length of the coaching and the training received was not provided. A nursing role (as coaching) to augment other interventions (education) is supported.
Driscoll, J., & Cooper, R. (2005). Coaching for clinicians. *Nursing Management, 12*(1), 18–22.	Coaching is a holistic term for the support of continuing personal and professional development. The clients' experiences and needs determine the degree to which coaching is directive or nondirective and may involve skills coaching, performance coaching, or development coaching. The ICF core competencies underpin the work of professional coaches. Professional coaching is an eclectic discipline based on knowledge from counseling, social sciences, neurolinguistics, management and business consulting, philosophy, and motivational psychology. It adopts an appreciative approach with clients. Key differences between coaching and clinical supervision are presented.

Appendix I

Dyess, S. M., Sherman, R., Opalinski, A., & Eggenberger, T. (2017). Structured coaching programs to develop staff. *The Journal of Continuing Education in Nursing, 48*(8), 373–378.	This article reflects on three coaching programs: Gallup Strengths-Based Coaching, Dartmouth Microsystem Coaching, and Health and Wellness Nurse Coaching. Each approach is presented, processes and outcomes are considered, and implications for educators are offered. Continuing education departments may recognize various coaching approaches as opportunities to support staff professionals achieve not only the triple aim, but also the quadruple aim.
Erickson, H. L., Erickson, M. E., Southard, M. E., Brekke, M. E., Sandor, M. K., & Natschke, M. (2016). A proactive innovation for health care transformation: Health and wellness nurse coaching. *Journal of Holistic Nursing, 34*(1), 44–55.	A cohort of holistic nurses, recognizing opportunities inherent in healthcare transformation, organized and worked together from 2009 to 2012. The goal was to hold space for holistic nursing by developing a health and wellness coaching role and certification program for holistic nurses. The American Holistic Credentialing Corporation's perspective of the events that unfolded and of the related decisions made by the coalition provides a record of the evolution of holistic nursing.
Erwin, D. M., & Vienneau, N. (2019). Battling burnout with nurse coaching: Stories from the ICU. *Beginnings, 39*(3), 16–17, 34.	This article explores how two critical care nurses learn nurse coaching strategies and incorporated the Theory of Integrative Nurse Coaching as a philosophical foundation for evidenced based practice. With their new awareness for self-compassion and setting healthy boundaries, they became more aware of healthy ways to manage stress and became more inspired as critical care nurses.

Fahey, K. F., Rao, S. M., Douglas, M. K., Thomas, M. L., Elliott, J. E., & Miaskowski, C. (2008). Nurse coaching to explore and modify patient attitudinal barriers interfering with effective cancer pain management. *Oncology Nursing Forum, 35*(2), 233–240.	Nurse coaching was used with patients with cancer pain to explore beliefs and attitudinal barriers interfering with pain management that included communication about pain management, and the use of analgesics and nonpharmacologic interventions. Nurse coaching reduced ineffective behaviors and improved pain treatment.
Fazio, S., Edwards, J., Miyamoto, S., Henderson, S., Dharmar, M., & Young, H. M. (2019). More than A1C: Types of success among adults with type-2 diabetes participating in a technology-enabled nurse coaching intervention. *Patient Education and Counseling, 102*(1), 106–112.	A qualitative analysis was conducted using surveys and documentation from motivational interview-based coaching sessions between study nurses and intervention participants. Of the 132 cases reviewed, types of success predominantly fell into five categories: 1) change in health behaviors; 2) change in mindset or awareness; 3) change in engagement with healthcare resources; 4) change in physical or emotional health; and 5) change in health indicators. The findings suggest coaching and technology can assist patients to achieve a range of successes in diabetes management through goal setting, health tracking, resolving barriers, and aligning goals with factors that impact change.

Appendix I

Fielden, S. L., Davidson, M. J., & Sutherland, V. J. (2009). Innovations in coaching and mentoring: Implications for nurse leadership development. *Health Services Management Research*, *22*(2), 92–99. doi: 10.1258/hsmr.2008.008021.	Coaching and mentoring are compared. Transformational coaching is a coaching process that involves development of rapport, relationship building, information gathering through assessment and review, negotiation of carefully defined goals, development of an action plan and implementation of problem solving. Coaching is not telling people what to do or how to do it. There are differences and similarities in coaching and mentoring. While mentoring was perceived to be "support" and coaching was described as "action," the actual process and content were quite similar. Mentoring may include aspects of coaching more than coaching incorporates aspects of mentoring.
Flinter, M., Hsu, C., Cromp, D. A., Ladden, M. J. D., & Wagner, E. H. (2017). Registered nurses in primary care: Emerging roles and contributions to team-based care in high-performing practices. *Journal of Ambulatory Care Management*, *40*(4), 287–96.	This study examined the roles of RNs in 30 exemplary primary care practices. They identified the emergence of new roles and activities for RNs characterized by greater involvement in face-to-face patient care and care management, their own daily schedule of patient visits and contacts, and considerable autonomy in the care of their patients.

Frey, L. M., & Ratliff, J. L. (2018). The personal and professional experiences of integrative nurse coach certificate program graduates: A pilot study. *Journal of Holistic Nursing, 36*(2), 134–144.	This qualitative pilot study (n = 13) describes Integrative Nurse Coach Certificate Program graduates' personal and professional experiences. Semistructured interviews identified the following common themes as follows: (1) development of self, (2) enriched self-care, (3) a call to action for facilitating the healthcare paradigm shift, and (4) incorporating Integrative Nurse Coaching into practice. The pilot study's findings and conclusions provide insight into the potential benefits of Integrative Nurse Coaching and the importance of nurse self-care.
Gortner, S. R., Gilliss, C. L., Shinn, J. A., Sparacino, P. A., Rankin, S., Leavitt, M., Price, M., & Hudes, M. (1988). Improving recovery following cardiac surgery: A randomized clinical trial. *Journal of Advanced Nursing, 13*, 649–661.	Nurses who provided a telephone monitoring intervention on post hospital cardiac surgery recovery and rehabilitation at home taught and coached on a variety of emotional and physical issues and assisted with problem solving. Master's and doctoral level nurses provided coaching. No set coaching protocol or training was discussed. No operational definition of coaching was provided.

Appendix I

Hayes, E., & Kalmakis, K. (2007). From the sidelines: Coaching as a nurse practitioner strategy for improving health outcomes. *Journal of the American Academy of Nurse Practitioners, 19*(11), 555–562.	The coaching process for nurse practitioners is described as method of developing "interpersonal communication skills" that promote the client's engagement in the health and wellness process. The client's needs, life experiences, and goals are the center of the relationship. The NP must be a good listener and assist the client in decision-making. Client characteristics are the driving force of the coaching interaction. Concepts can be applied to nurses in a variety of roles other than NP. This approach also supports the transtheoretical stages of change model and motivational interviewing techniques.
Heath, J., Kelley, F. J., Andrews, J., Crowell, N. et al. (2007). Evaluation of a tobacco cessation curricular intervention among acute care nurse practitioner faculty members. *American Journal of Critical Care, 16*(3), 284–289.	Nurse coaching is expanding and NPs need to have tools that can assist tobacco users in deciding to stop. There is an opportunity to add nurse coaching to educational nursing programs.
Heckerson, E. W. (2006, February). Nurse leader as coach. *Nurse Leader, 4*(1), 29–31.	Nurses are natural coaches and coaching is an inherent responsibility of nurse leaders. High-performing leaders focus on coaching. Essential attributes of a coach are passion, integrity, energy, creativity, and excellent communication. Coaching strategies include asking question, listening carefully without judgment, considering all options, offering specific constructive, direct, and supportive feedback, and building on strengths. Open dialogue and a relationship of mutual trust are essential. Nurse coaching is an exciting new role for the 21st century.

Hennessey, B., & Suter, P. (2011). The community-based transitions model: One agency's experience. *Home Healthcare Nurse, 29*(4), 218–230.	Transitional care is a central part of the Patient Protection and Affordable Care Act of 2010. CMS is working with states to design, implement, and evaluate care transition improvement programs. One model involves the use of a health coach—one who abandons the traditional role of "doing" for the patient in favor of role modeling self-care. Another model utilizes advanced practice nurse as transition coaches. Common characteristics necessary for health coaches are presented. Health coach is a term that is not uniformly defined, but may include home health nurses as coaches—a role that is compatible with professional nursing practice and requires minimal retooling.
Hess, D., Bark, L., & Southard, M. E. (2010, September). White paper: Holistic Nurse Coaching. *Summit on standards & credentialing of professional coaches in healthcare & wellness.*	Paper presented to National Credentialing Team for Professional Coaches in Healthcare, Boston, MA. Retrieved March 1, 2012 from http://www.ahncc.org/holisticnurse-coaching.html

Appendix I

Hess, D. R., Dossey, B. M., Southard, M. E., Luck, S., Schaub, B. G., & Bark, L. (2013). *The art and science of nurse coaching: A provider's guide to coaching scope and competencies.* Silver Spring, MD: Nursesbooks.org.	This document describes the rapidly emerging role of the nurse coach that is grounded in the principles and core values of professional nursing. Nurse coaching competencies can be integrated into any setting or specialty area of practice. It is a structured, relationship-centered approach by RNs promotes achievement of client goals, and the interactions with clients are skilled, purposeful, and results-oriented. Nurse coaches establish cocreative partnerships with clients to facilitate a process of change and realize undeveloped potential. It contains the foundational criteria and a process for the American Holistic Nurses Credentialing Corporation Nurse Coach certification exam (i.e., educational training, content, skills, practice hours, supervision and testing organization/certification titles).
Higgins, K., & Scott, M. A. (2019). Using health coaching to improve patients' BP management. *Nursing, 49*(6), 44–48. doi: 10.1097/01. NURSE.0000554245.67012.03.	This article describes the use of health coaching to help patients understand their medications and give them the knowledge, skills, and confidence to self-manage their hypertension. Nurses have unique opportunities to influence patient outcomes and reduce healthcare expenditures. Health coaching is one patient-centered strategy nurses can use to improve the limited health literacy often associated with hypertension.
Huffman, M. (2007). Health coaching: A new and exciting technique to enhance patient self-management and improve outcomes. *Home Healthcare News, 25*(4), 271–274.	Health coaching is described as a partnering with clients to enhance self-management. Medicare pilot testing this approach for patients with CHF and DM.

Jackson, K., D'Avolio, & Gropper, S. (2019). Choosing coaching frameworks for promoting diet modifications. *British Journal of Nursing, 28*(22), 1456–1560.	Theoretical frameworks have successfully guided researches in implementing coaching interventions to effect dietary changes in adults for both prevention and management of chronic diseases. Three such frameworks include the Transtheoretical Model (TMM), Social Cognitive Theory (SCT), and the Theory of Integrative Nurse Coaching (TINC). This article introduces each theory, followed by an overview of the coaching interventions used to effect dietary behavior changes within each theory.
Johnson, V. D. (2007). Promoting behavior change: Making healthy choices in wellness and healing choices in illness—Use of self-determination theory in nursing practice. *Nursing Clinics of North America, 42*(2), 229–241.	Holistic nurses can use Self-Determination Theory (SDT) to promote healthy behavior change. As nurses act in ways to support clients' innate needs for autonomy, competence, and relatedness, clients may be more successful at internalizing self-regulation and more incline to adopt and maintain life-long behavioral changes.
Jones, D., Dufy, M. E., & Flanagan, J. (2011). Randomized clinical trial testing efficacy of a nurse-coached intervention in arthroscopy patients. *Nursing Research, 60*(2), 92–99.	The nurse-coached intervention "focused on giving information, interpreting the experience, and validating and clarifying responses and actions related to the surgical experience directed toward making a difference in recovery outcomes" (p. 93). Nurse coaches received three 2-hr classes related to the study. The coaching intervention was delivered by telephone. Nurse coaches were provided with clinical guidelines and a set of questions to guide the discussion with the patient.

Appendix I

Kelly, M., & Starr, T. (2008). From hospital to home: An innovative program eases discharged patients back into the community. *Advance for Nurses*, 5(18), 12.	Senior level BSN students provided coaching based on the Coleman Transition Intervention, a method designed to promote client empowerment and self-advocacy skills through a coaching intervention model. "As today's healthcare paradigm shifts patients toward shared decision making with their providers, the next generation of nurses will need specific competencies that facilitate their clients" empowerment of their personal healthcare management" (p. 1).
Kelly, J., Crowe, P., & Shearer, M. (2005). The Good Life Project: Telephone coaching for chronic disease self management. *Australian Family Physician*, 34(1–2), 31–34.	Coaching was provided monthly over 12 months by student nurses to promote client empowerment and self-advocacy skills through the use of a coaching intervention model. Coaches received 2 days of motivational interviewing training that also included identifying depression, anxiety, and levels of social support in participants. Patients were specifically encouraged to adhere to recommended treatment.

Lenzen, S. A., Daniëls, R., van Bokhoven, M. A., van der Weijden, T., & Beurskens, A. (2018). What makes it so difficult for nurses to coach patients in shared decision-making? A process evalua-tion. *International Journal of Nursing Studies, 80,* 1–11.	This process evaluation was con-ducted using quantitative and qual-itative methods to investigate how the coaching approach was imple-mented and experienced by practice nurses and patients. Fifteen female practice nurses (aged between 28 and 55 years), working with peo-ple suffering from diabetes, COPD, asthma, and/or cardiovascular diseases, participated. Nurses were asked to apply the approach to their chronically ill patients and to recruit patients (n = 10) willing to partic-ipate in an interview or an audio recording of a consultation (n = 13); patients (13 women, 10 men) were aged between 41 and 88 years and suffered from diabetes, COPD or cardiovascular diseases. Overall, nurses felt that the approach sup-ported them to coach patients in shared decision making. However, nurses struggled to integrate the approach in routine care.
Manne, S. L., Bakeman, R., Jacobsen, P. B., Gorfinkle, K., & Redd, W. H. (1994). An analysis of a behavioural intervention for children undergoing venipuncture. *Health Psychology, 13*(6), 556–566.	Nurse coaches received 1 hr of training on how to properly coach parents while their child (ages 36–107 months) experienced veni-puncture. The nurse coached par-ents to encourage the child to use a party blower and to verbally help them through the procedure.

Appendix I

McElligott, D., Eckardt, S., Dossey, B. M., Luck, S., & Eckardt, P. (2018). Instrument development of integrative health and wellness assessments. *Journal of Holistic Nursing, 36*(4), 374–384.	This article describes the history of the Integrative Health and Wellness Assessment (IHWA) tool and the development and pilot testing of the IHWA short form. The Theory of Integrative Nurse Coaching provides a foundation for coaching interventions and the development of the IHWA short form. This 36-question Likert-type scale self-reporting tool assists participants in assessing healthy behaviors through a self-reflection process, provides information for the coaching relationship, and may be an outcome measurement.
McElligott, D. (2014). Innovations in holistic nursing: The role of the nurse coach. *Beginnings, 34*(8), 26–28.	The innovative role of nurse coach, clearly identified and grounded in theory, must be supported with evidence-based practice and ongoing research. Data collection and validation tools are needed to demonstrate the value and effectiveness of nurse coaching. Additional research validating the benefits of nurse coaching will open doors for nurses to practice to the fullest extent of their role as holistic nurses, maintain a viable income, and become a valued part of the interprofessional team.
McNally, K., & Cunningham, L. (2010). *The Nurse Executive's Coaching Manual.* Indianapolis, IN: Sigma Theta Tau International.	This coaching manual is for nurse executives. It provides an overview of the coaching approach, competencies, models, tools, and resources that will be applicable to coaching other leaders in a healthcare organization. Coaching is a learning and development strategy that provides the leader with the tools necessary to enhance individual and organizational performance, support succession planning, and help future leaders make successful transitions.

Medland, J., & Stern, M. (2009). Coaching as a successful strategy for advancing new manager competency and performance. *Journal of Nurses Staff Development, 25*(3), 141–147.	Employing the expertise of a dedicated coach is a unique approach to advance competency of new nurse managers in the formative stage of development. This article describes how coaching is emerging as an essential tool for new manager development.
Miller, C. (2011). An integrated approach to worker self-management and health outcomes: Chronic conditions, evidence-based practice, and health coaching. *American Association of Occupational Health Nurses, 59*(11), 491–501.	Occupational health nursing practice will be impacted by the new trends in health coaching, evidence-based practice, and standards of care. Occupational health nurses posses the scientific knowledge related to acute and chronic disease symptoms, stress-management, relationships. By incorporating new health coaching skills they can assist employees to learn self-discovery and self-management that have the potential to produce optimal health outcomes.
Mitchell, G. J., Cross, N., Wilson, M., Biernacki, W. W., Adib, B., & Rush, D. (2013). Complexity and health coaching: Synergies in nursing. *Nursing Research & Practice.* Article ID238620. http://dx.doi.org/10.1155/2013/238620.	Human beings are complex and are living in complex systems and evolving in nonlinear ways and are influenced by the systems in which they live. Informed by complexity science, the RN Health Coach (RNHC) role is a creative innovation in community settings to care for people with acute and chronic illnesses. This article explores complexity science and its implication for the RNHC role.

Appendix I

Miyamoto, S., Dharmar, M., Fazio, S., Feldman, Y. T., Heather, M., & Young, H. M. (2018). mHealth technology and nurse health coaching to improve health in diabetes: Protocol for a randomized controlled trial. *Journal of Medical Internet Research Protocols, 7*(2), e45, doi:10.2196/resprot.9168.	This clinical trial evaluated the impact of a mobile health (mHealth) enabled nurse health coaching intervention on self-efficacy among adults with type-2 diabetes mellitus. This randomized controlled trial was conducted at an academic health system in Northern California. A total of 300 participants with type-2 diabetes were scheduled to be enrolled through three primary care clinics. This protocol details a patient-centered intervention using nurse health coaching, mHealth technologies, and integration of patient-generated data into the EHR. The aim of the intervention is to enhance self-efficacy and health outcomes by providing participants with a mechanism to track daily activity by offering coaching support to set reasonable and attainable health goals, and by creating a complete feedback loop by bringing patient-generated data into the EHR.
Mott, M. (1992). Cognitive coaching for nurse educators. *The Journal of Nursing Education, 31*(4), 188–190.	Coaching model is described as peer cognitive coaching to enhance faculty development and thus student achievement. Coaching involves positive feedback to enhance and reinforce desired behavior. The model allows for personal and professional growth through trust, openness, and curiosity. Discussion and critique of others' views are promoted.

Naylor, M., & Keating, S. A. (2008). Transitional care. *Journal of Social Work Education*, Supplement, *44*(3), 65–73.	Nurse-led multidisciplinary transitions care models that engage the patient and caregivers in discharge planning have consistently improved quality and cost-savings. One intervention model described as care transition coaching encourages older patients and family caregivers to assume more active roles during care transitions. An advanced practice nurse serves as a "transitions coach" to engage, teach, and promote cross-site continuity of care. Coaching begins in hospital and for 30 days after discharge. Available studies indicate that a focus on patient and caregiver needs, preferences, and goals is one of four key elements of improving care transition.
Niesen, C. R., Kraft, S. J., & Meiers, S. J. (2018). Use of motivational interviewing by nurse leaders: Coaching for performance, professional development, and career goal setting. *The Health Care Manager*, *37*(2), 183–192.	This article describes motivational interviewing (MI) as a mentoring style to guide patients toward health promotion and disease management. The aims of this project were (1) to identify evidence supporting the application of MI strategies and principles by nurse leaders to promote healthful leadership development among direct-report staff and (2) to report outcomes of an educational pilot project regarding MI use for new nurse leaders. Correlations between MI and the American Organization of Nurse Executives nurse executive competencies are reviewed and summarized. The results show acceptability for MI use in professional development of direct-report staff and in other aspects of nursing leadership roles.

Appendix I

Old, N. (2012). Positive health coaching: the way forward in nursing. *Australian Nursing Journal, 20*(2), 32.	Nursing is moving into new phase of health delivery that involves assisting clients to increase healthy behaviors. A nurse coach model of care is described. A nurse coach supports people to develop the skills of self-awareness to achieve their health goals. Self-empowerment is encouraged. Nurse coaches focus on client perspectives, expectations, and specific concerns. The Transtheoretical Model, positive psychology, and a focus on client motivation and on what is working rather than what is not, provide frameworks for successful nurse coaching.
Ponte, P. R., Gross, A., H., Galante, A., & Glazer, G. (2006). Using an executive coach to increase leadership effectiveness. *Journal of Nursing Administration, 36*(6), 319–324.	Engaging a leadership coach is a trend and being used as innovative nursing leadership self-development programs and practices. Reporting on four coaches and four nurse leaders, this article reports on the effectiveness of coaching as a leadership development tool and make recommendations for leaders interested in engaging a coach.
Potempa, K. M., Butterworth, S. W., Flaherty-Robb, M. K., & Gaynor, W. L. (2010). The Healthy Ageing Model: Health behaviour change for older adults. *Collegian: Royal College of Nursing, Australia, 17*(2), 51–55.	The Healthy Ageing Model focuses on aging adults and has four elements—client-centered, goal-driven approach, individualized coaching strategy of behavioral change, and personal health system. Care is delivered by a nurse practitioner or a primary care physician via in-person clinic visits or home visits, telephone, or e-mail. Behavioral coaching is the core strategy with the ongoing shift to a client-centered relationship of health promotion with the coach as the client's support partner.

Radtke, K. (2019). Advanced nurse coaching in patients with complex needs. *Beginnings, 39*(1), 22–23.	This article explores the journey of a holistic nurse practitioner and nurse coach working with patients with multiple comorbid and complex needs. Tips for working with complex needs are provided. The importance of integrating research and evidence-based practice is discussed.
Rivers, R., Pesata, V., Beasley, M., & Dietrich, M. (2011, October). Transformational leadership: Creating a prosperity-planning coaching model for RN retention. *Nurse Leader, 9*(5), 48–51.	To assist nurses to develop resilience to the effects of compassion stress, 30 nurse managers and staff nurses enrolled in a 20-week program with a life coach. All who completed the program viewed it as a positive experience and indicated that the most helpful aspect was having a consistent, nonjudgmental person to provide feedback and suggestions. An overall theme of self-awareness was noted by participants. Improved resilience and retention indicators were evident.

Appendix I

Ross, A., Brooks, A. T., Yang, L., Touchton-Leonard, K., Raju, S., & Bevans, M. (2018). Results of a national survey of certified nurse coaches with implications for advanced practice nurses. *Journal of the American Association of Nurse Practitioners, 30*(5), 251–261.	This study describes the practices of nurse coaches including their work settings, clients/health conditions, and motivations behind becoming certified as coaches, and the personal benefits experienced by nurse coaches. A cross-sectional online survey was e-mailed to certified nurse coaches (n = 315) with 164 completing the survey; it included 68 (41.5%) advanced practice nurses. Coaching varied in frequency, method (individual versus group), mode (in-person, by phone, or electronically). Results showed that participants became coaches to gain skills for enhancing their practice, to deliver care that fits with their values and philosophy, to meet personal needs (starting a private practice and improve their own self-care), attaining credentials/validation, and to empower others. The majority agreed/strongly agreed that since becoming a nurse coach, their own interpersonal relationships (80.3%), health/health behaviors (84.8%), and job satisfaction (70.7%) improved.
Samarel, N., Fawcett, J., & Tulman. (1997). Effect of support groups with coaching on adaptation to early state breast cancer. *Research in Nursing & Health, 20*(1), 15–26.	A nurse/social worker team referred to as "expert clinicians" led coaching support groups. The coaches were significant others of participants. No formal definition of coaching was provided. Clinician team training consisted of a 4-hour training session with a manual for them to follow.

Schaub, B. G., & White, M. B. (2015). Transpersonal coaching. *Beginnings, 35*(4), 24–25.	This article shares the benefit nurses and patients can gain from transpersonal coaching. This practice blends well with holistic nursing, nurse coaching, and can be easily applied to a variety of situations and healthcare settings. As the nurse explores the transpersonal aspect of human nature the individual may gain access to her or his transpersonal nature and thereby experience new feelings and insights that usually come in the form of images and energies and provide the personality with a greater sense of wholeness and courage.
Schaub, B. G., Luck, S., & Dossey, B. (2012). Integrative nurse coaching for health and wellness. *Alternative and Complementary Therapies, 18*(1), 14–20.	The Samueli Institute in its Wellness Initiative for the Nation recommended the education of health and wellness coaches to improve the nation's healthcare system by changing to a wellness model. This recommendation was written into the PPACA law. This article addresses the implementation of this transition through the development of the nurse coach role. Professional nurse coaches are in every healthcare setting and are ideally positioned to take leading roles in implementing new models of care that emphasize health and wellness. Integrative nursing principles and the Integrative Nurse Coach Model are described. The Theory of Integral Nursing is presented as a framework for integrative nurse coaching.

Appendix I

Schenak, S. (2002). Nurse coaching: Healthcare resource for this millennium. *Nursing Forum, 37*(3), 16–20.	Nurse coaching is described as a new role for nurses. It is client-directed as opposed to illness-directed. The nurse coach can provide a structure and an approach with the patient/client to custom fit toward attainable behavioral change. Specific aspects of the nurse coach role include integration of self-efficacy, promoting lifestyle changes, readiness for change, and motivation.
Sethares, K. A. (2003). Supporting the self-care behaviors of women with heart failure through an individualized nursing intervention (Doctoral dissertation) Boston College, Boston, MA). Available from *Dissertation Abstracts Online* (363).	Coaching was provided by an advance practice nurse and followed the Individualized Nursing Care Model of Self-care for Women with heart failure. Coaching was used to educate and support. The nurse coach visited each participant (n = 7) for 1 h once per week for 4 weeks. Each session was audio taped.
Southard, M. E. (2003). An integrative approach to wellness coaching: emerging standards of nurse coaching practice. Copyright.	Based on holistic philosophy and nursing theory, this model for health and wellness coaching provides the framework for nurse coaching education and practice.
Southard, M. E. (2015). The nuances of cultural diversity in coaching. *Beginnings, 35*(4), 22–23.	This article explores the significance of an individual's' cultural beliefs and rituals on health choices and behaviors. It discusses the impact of culture on diet, healthcare practices, and the Health Belief Model based on culture. It focuses on the importance of recognizing an individual's values and beliefs and how the nurse coach can engage one's cultural diversity for creative solutions toward health and well-being.

Southard, M. E., Bark, L., Erickson, M., & Monsen, K. A. (2017). Feasibility of using the Omaha System to represent Nurse Coaching practice. *Kontakt, 19*(1), e4–e11.	Nurse coaching is an important strategy for improving the health of populations. Effective interventions for nurse coaching (NC) practice, fair value outcome measurements, and standardization of terms have yet to be determined. As healthcare systems adopt electronic medical records and as nurse coaching practice evolves, it is important to capture and identify NC interventions. The long-term goal is to improve patient-centered practice by using standardized interface terminology and to examine the feasibility of using the Omaha System to represent NC practice. The three aims were to evaluate content validity of NC case studies, test accuracy of NC graduates identifying Omaha System terms for NC interventions, and explore the feasibility of analyzing NC case study data.
Stefancyk, A., Hancock, B., & Meadows, M. T. (2013). The nurse manager: Change agent, change coach? *Nursing Administration Quarterly, 37*(1), 13–17.	A change coach, building upon the nurse manager's foundations skill of coaching, uses coaching skills to inspire others toward change. Being a change coach reflects the art of change that includes mobilizing the resources toward innovation and improvement. Three categories of coaching behavior are discussed: guidance, facilitation, and inspiration. Change coaching is viewed as a leadership imperative and a skill needed by successful nurse managers. A greater emphasis on coaching to influence change requires further development to expand the skills and behaviors of all nurse leaders.

Appendix I

Stewart-Lord, A., Baillie, L., & Woods, S. (2017). Health care staff perceptions of a coaching and mentoring programme: A qualitative case study evaluation. *International Journal of Evidence Based Coaching and Mentoring, 15*(2), 70–85.	This study aimed to determine the value of the Coaching and Mentoring (C&M) Programme within a large National Health Service (NHS) system ("Trust") in London, England. A case study design was utilized with units of analysis: mentors, mentees, coaches, coachees, and line managers. Semistructured interviews (n = 32) took place in 2015. Findings revealed how individuals were able to develop personally and professionally. Findings support the need for more staff opportunities to engage in shared activities. The study also identified the importance of there being strong organization-wide leadership of the program, as well as managerial support to enable staff to engage in the program.
Stuart-Mullen, L., Cutshall, S., Wentworth, L., & Loth, A. (2015). Bringing nurse coaching to a cardiovascular health clinic. *Beginnings, 35*(4), 6–9.	A pilot offering introductory nurse coaching education was initiated with a small group of Cardiovascular Health Clinic (CVHC) nurses at a large Midwest medical center. A plan was established to provide training during the lunch hour for four nonconsecutive days. The training included 12 CVHC nurses completing this course. Feedback regarding the training course was solicited via a pre and post evaluation survey. The report showed that the small training cohort report were now taking a new approach to the process of goal identification for their cardiac rehabilitation patients.

Sullivan, V. H., & Hays, M. M., & Alexander, S. (2019). Health coaching for patients with type 2 diabetes mellitus to decrease 30-day hospital readmissions. *Professional Case Management, 24*(2), 76–82. doi: 10.1097/ NCM.0000000000000304.	The purpose of this program was to provide health coaching to patients with a primary or secondary diagnosis of Type 2 diabetes mellitus (T2DM) to increase self-management skills and reduce 30-day readmissions. The setting was a 273-bed, acute care not-for-profit hospital in the southern region of the United States. The majority of patients reported accomplishment of goals with 16 out of 20 patients who did not require inpatient stay 30 days after discharge from the acute care facility. The T2DM piloted program can easily be modified to fit other chronic illness that require routine monitoring and complex regimens to remain healthy. Case managers have the opportunity to coach on the importance of lifestyle modification and self-management support for patients with chronic illness with follow-up interactive phone visits after hospital discharge.
Stulbarg, M. S., Carrieri-Kohlman, V., Gormley, J. M., Tsang, A., & Paul, S. (1999). Accuracy of recall of dyspnea after exercise training sessions. *Journal of Cardiopulmonary Rehabilitation, 19*(4), 242–248.	A master's prepared nurse coach provided the coaching. At the beginning of each coaching session, the nurse coach helped participants (n = 44) set goals related to their clinical status. Coaching was based on guided mastery techniques that included vicarious experiences, verbal persuasion, and physiological feedback.

Appendix I

Sutters, K. A., Miaskowski, C., Holdridge-Zeuner, D., Waite, S., Paul, S. M., Savedra, M., & Lanier, B. (2004). A randomized clinical trial of the effectiveness of a scheduled oral analgesic dosing regimen for the management of postoperative pain in children following tonsillectomy. *Pain, 110*(1–2), 49–55.	A research nurse provided nurse coaching via telephone calls to parents on days 1 and 2 post surgery that consisted of an evaluation of the child's condition, review of pain intensity, verification that the child was taking the medication, re-education of the rationale for the dosing, review of strategies to give the medication to the child, and repeat education concerning potential side effects of the medication. One nurse coach delivered the same information during all the coaching calls to maintain consistency.
Sutters, K. A., Miaskowski, C., Holdridge-Zeuner, D., Waite, S., Paul, S. M., Savedra, M., & Lanier, B. (2005). Time-contingent dosing of an opioid analgesic after tonsillectomy does not increase moderate-to-severe side effects in children. *Pain Management Nursing, 6*(2), 49–57.	A research nurse provided nursing coaching via telephone calls to parents on days 1 and 2 post surgery that consisted of a discussion of postoperative pain experiences, an explanation of the administration of a nonopioid with an opioid analgesic, a review of the ordered dosing regimen, strategies for improving adherence, teaching regarding possible side effects, and an explanation about myths about psychological addiction. The nurse also evaluated the child's condition, reviewed pain levels, and verified the child was taking the medication. One nurse coach delivered the same information during all the coaching calls to maintain consistency.

Tidwell, L., Holland, S., Greenberg, J., Malone, J., Mullan, J., & Newcomer, R. (2004). Community-based nurse health coaching and its effect on fitness participation. *Lippincott's Case Management, 9*(6), 267–279.	Coaching was part of a program provided by a nurse coach, a social worker, and a geriatrician that included using a client developed health action plan, patient education instruction and classes, and a fitness program to increase physical activity. A focus was to improve chronic disease self-management, and improve self-confidence in communicating with a primary care provider. Nurse coaching was used to empower participants (504 members of the California Public Employees Retirement system) through encouragement to make healthy choices toward healthier way of living as outlined by the Case Management Society of America. The nurse coach provided health education, counseling, and medication management coaching. The article did not report how each participant was coached.
van Houwelingen, C. T., Moerman, A. H., Ettema, R. G., Kort, H. S., & ten Cate, O. (2016). Competencies required for nursing telehealth activities: A Delphi-study. *Nurse Education Today, 39,* 50–62.	In a four-round Delphi-study, a panel of experts discussed which nursing telehealth entrustable professional activities (NT-EPAs) are relevant for nurses and which competencies nurses need to possess in order to execute these activities effectively. The threshold used for consensus was set at 80%. In total, 52 competencies were identified essential in telehealth. Additionally, the 14 NT-EPAs appeared to require additional subject specific competencies, such as the ability to put patients at ease when they feel insecure about using technology.

Appendix I

Vale, M., Jelinek, M., Grigg, L., & Newman, R. (2003). Coaching patients on achieving cardiovascular health (COACH). *Archives of Internal Medicine, 163*(22), 2775–2783.	The coaches for this program were four nurses and two dieticians that were hospital based. The coaches used telephone calls and mailings to coach patients. Coaches underwent two weeks of part-time coaching training using the COACH model developed by the authors.
Vienneau, N. (2018). Nurse coaches are essential to healing the health-care industry. *Multibriefs*, May 25. http://exclusive.multibriefs.com/content/nurse-coaches-are-essential-to-healing-the-healthcare-industry/healthcare-administration.	Nurse coaches blend the art and science of health and well-being into practice. The nurse coach journey of authentic presence is developed. It illustrates how nurse coaches cocreate a space that honors a person's essence. Examples are given to show ways the healthcare system can be healed and changed with nurse coaches.
Vincent, A. E., & Sanchez Birkhead, A. C. (2013). Evaluation of the effectiveness of nurse coaching in improving health outcomes in chronic conditions. *Holistic Nursing Practice, 27*(3), 148–61.	Nurse coaching was explored as a legitimate, holistic enhancement to Western medicine. Thirteen research studies were reviewed and outcomes discussed that were related to nurse coaching interventions in patients with various chronic conditions. All but two of these studies reported at least some statistically significant positive health outcomes.
Vojta, D., De Sa, J., Prospect, T., & Stevens, S. (2012). Effective interventions for stemming the growing crisis of diabetes and prediabetes: A national payer's perspective. *Health Affairs, 31*(1), 20–26.	New evidence-based consumer care models that support and encourage lifestyle changes for those with diabetic conditions include partnerships with pharmacists, nurses, and health coaches. Health plans are participating in projects designed to dramatically impact diabetes risk through carefully tailored lifestyle interventions led by lifestyle coaches.

Waldrop, J., & Derouin, A. (2019). The coaching experience of advanced practice nurses in a national leadership program. *Journal of Continuing Education in Nursing, 50*(4), 170. doi: 10.3928/00220124-20190319-07.	This article describes describe the current literature related to coaching among APNs and the results of this coaching experience. Coaching circles are a technique used in the Duke-Johnson & Johnson Nurse Leadership Program to provide guidance and expertise to small groups of advanced practice nurse (APN).
	A serial cross-sectional survey design was used to evaluate the coaching circle experience of four cohorts of Fellows from 2013–2017. Evidence in the literature related to the use of coaching specifically among APNs is limited. Participants evaluated the structure and function, as well as the value, of the coaching circle. This report offers insight into strategies of coaching that would be useful in a variety of healthcare settings to promote the advancement of nurse leaders.
Ward, A. M. (2018). I wish I had a school nurse like you. *Beginnings, 38*(3), 10–11.	This article discusses how a school nurse uses nurse coaching and integrates imagery, centering, and energy healing techniques with transpersonal coaching skills to reduce the many manifestations of anxiety among grade school children. It also focuses on the importance of the school nurse practicing self-reflection in order to be fully present to support the students in their emotional/mental/social needs.

Appendix I

Whittemore, R. (2000). A coaching intervention to integrate lifestyle change in adults with non-insulin dependent diabetes mellitus (Doctoral dissertation, Boston College, 2000). *Dissertation Abstracts Online*, 285.	Participants (n = 9) received eight weeks of nurse coaching aimed at facilitating diabetes self-care patients' existing lifestyle. Four coaching sessions were completed throughout the 8-week period and each session was in-person for approximately 60 min. Coaching was used to educate, support, and provide guidance to participants. How the coaching was implemented was not described.
Whittemore, R., Chase, S. K., Mandle, C. L., & Roy, C. (2002). Lifestyle change in type 2 diabetes. *Nursing Research, 51*(1), 18–25.	The nurse coaching model used for this study was a modified version of the Adaptation of Chronic Illness Model. Nurse coaching consisted of: providing diabetes information; identifying barriers and facilitators to lifestyle change; providing motivational support; giving feedback and positive encouragement; and goal setting. Nurse coaching was delivered by an advanced practice nurse and consisted of individual four 45-min sessions every 2 weeks.
Whittemore, R., D'Eramo Melkus, G., Sullivan, A., & Grey, M. (2004). A nurse-coaching intervention for women with type 2 diabetes. *The Diabetes Educator, 30*(5), 795–804.	A nurse coach provided coaching to educate, assist, and provide support to increase maintenance of patient self-management. Participants (n = 49) received six personal coaching sessions, using a coaching model developed by the primary author (and others), over a 6-month period. It was not clear how the coaching was done.

Wilkie, D. J., Williams, A. R., Grevstad, P., & Mekwa, J. (1995). Coaching persons with lung cancer to report sensory pain: Literature review and pilot study findings. *Cancer Nursing, 18*(1).	Coaching was defined as a method for patients to become more educated and active in their own pain management. Coaching was an interactive process that assumed patients are active processors of information, can elicit beliefs and attitudes to promote change, can learn more adoptive ways of thinking, feeling, and behaving, and be active in their own behavior change. Patients in the coached group were instructed how to self-monitor pain, how to qualify the pattern and intensity of their pain, and how to best report the pain to a clinician. This information was reinforced 1 week later during a telephone call.
Zhang, P., Hu, Y. D., Xing, F. M., Li, C. Z., Lan, W. F., & Zhang, X. L. (2017). Effects of a nurse-led transitional care program on clinical outcomes, health-related knowledge, physical and mental health status among Chinese patients with coronary artery disease: A randomized controlled trial. *International Journal of Nursing Studies, 74*, 34–43.	Effects of a nurse-led transitional care program on clinical outcomes, health related knowledge, physical and mental health status among Chinese patients with coronary artery disease. A randomized control trial.

Index

A

abuse, in nurse coaching, 25, 45

accountability, in nurse coaching, 10, 25, 60

active imagination, defined, 85, appA.180

acute care settings, in nurse coaching, 47

adaptation model (Roy), 21

administrators, 39, appA. 129, appA. 133, appA.136

advanced practice nurses (APRNs), 39, 47, 48–49, 52, 66, appA.136. *See also* graduate and advanced practice nurse coach, competencies

advocacy, in nurse coaching, 18, 24

aesthetic knowing, 87, appB.216

Aetna, 56–57

alcohol consumption, appA.155
  mortality and morbidity, 54

ambulatory care nurses, 39, appA.136

American Association of Colleges of Nursing (AACN), 53

American Holistic Nurses Credentialing Corporation (AHNCC), 9, 51

American Holistic Nurses Credentialing Corporation (AHNCC) nurse coach certification process
  certification examination development, appE.239–240
  nurse coach certification credentials, 51, appE.240
  nusing alliances, initiating, appE.239

American Nurses Credentialing Center (ANCC), 9

American Organization of Nurse Executives (AONE), 46, 61

America's great outdoors initiative, appA.157

Antonovsky, A.—*Sense-of-Coherence Theory,* 23, appA.221, appC.234

anxiety, in nurse coaching, 14, 45, 47, 65

appreciative inquiry (AI) (Cooperrider and Whitney), 22, appC.225–226

art and science, incorporation of, appA.135

The Art and Science of Nurse Coaching, appA.134, appA.140, appA.145, appA.147–148, appA.173, appA.177

client-centered goals, appA.134
  achievement of, appA.138
  cultural relevance, appA.135
  empowerment and motivation, appA.138
  establishing, appA.138. *See also person-centered goals.*
client-nurse relationship, appA.146, appA.148
client's agenda, appA.135
client's vulnerability, appA.153
clinical competency, in nurse coaching, 52–53
clinical decision-making, in nurse coaching, 13
clinical nurse leaders (CNL), 44
clinical setting, in nurse coaching, 39
clinics, nurse coaches practice, 13
coach, defined, 50, appA.147. *See also* nurse coach(es)
Coaching in Nursing, appA.149
coaching interaction, appA.134–135
  creating structure, appA.138
  nurse-client, appA.139
coaching model (Bark), appA.149
code of ethics, appA.153
Code of Ethics for Nurses with Interpretive Statements, 1, 14, 23, appA.170
codes, in nurse coaching, 57
coherence, in nurse coaching, 14
collaboration, 11, 19, 24, 26–27, 29, 48, 56, 64
  competencies, 80, appA. 176
  Standards of Professional Practice, appA.141
collaborative health planning and intervention, in nurse coaching, 64
commitment, in nurse coaching, 15, 24, 25, 30
communicable disease, appA.155

communication, 4, 10, 23, 32, 33–34, 40–41, 60, 61, 66, appA.153
  competencies, 79–80, appA. 141, appA. 174
  direct, 60, 75–76, appA.166–168
communication skills, 40, 60, 76, appA.138
communities, in nurse coaching, 14, 20, 24, 39, 42–44
community setting, in nurse coaching, 39
compassion, in nurse coaching, 16, 23–24, 34
compassion fatigue (CF), in nurse coaching, 47
competencies,
  assessment, 72, appA. 141, appA.159–160, appH. 253–254
  collaboration, 80, appA.176
  communication, 79, appA.174
  culturally congruent practice, 79, appH. 260
  diagnosis, 72–73, appA. 161
  education, 81, appA.171
  environmental health, 84, appA.179
  ethics, 78–79, appA.170
  evaluation, 78, appA. 169
  evidence-based practice and research, 81–82, appA.172
  implementation, 73–78, appA.164–168
  leadership, 80–81, appA.175
  outcomes identification, 73, appA.162
  planning, 73, appA.163
  professional practice evaluation, 83, appA.177
  quality of practice, 82, appA.173
  resource utilization, 84, appA.178
competencies in nurse coaching, 14, 21, 25, 26–27, appA.153
  assurance of, appA.142
  clinical, 52–53

defined, appA.142
evaluation, 53, appA.144
Complexity Science (Langeland, Wahl,
Kristoffersen, and Hanestad;
Chenowth, Gallagher, Sheriff,
Donoghue, and Stein-Parbury), 22
comprehensibility, appC.234
confidence, in nurse coaching, 21
confidentiality, in nurse coaching,
24–25
conflict, in nurse coaching, 35
consciousness, appA.151
continuous quality improvement, in
nurse coaching, 13
Cooperrider, David and Diana
Whitney—Appreciative Inquiry,
22, appA.210, appC. 225–226
coordinating care, in nurse coaching,
40, 64
core values, nurse coaching, 14,
19–39
coronary heart disease (CHD), risk
for, 44, 45
courtesy, in nurse coaching, 21
Cowling, Richard, 22
unitary appreciative inquiry,
appA.210, appB.223
unitary knowing in nursing
practice, appB.220
CPT codes, 66
creativity, in nurse coaching, 14, 15
credibility, in nurse coaching, 21
critical reasoning, in nurse coaching, 18
critical thinking, 18, appA.135
Csikszentmihalyi, Mihaly, *See*
Seligman, Martin and Mihaly
Csikszentmihalyi
cultural competence, in nurse
coaching, 37
culturally congruent practice, in
nurse coaching, 4, 37, 79, AppH.
260

culture, in nurse coaching, 12, 13,
18, 23–24, appA.135
customs, in nurse coaching, 37
CVS, 56–57

D

data management, in nurse coaching,
39, 63
Deci, Edward, 22, appC.227
deep listening, appA.165
defined, appA.180
dementia, in nurse coaching, 43
depression, in nurse coaching, 43,
45, 54
diabetes education, in nurse
coaching, 39
diagnosis, 31, 32, 72, appA. 137–
138, appA. 141, appA. 161
DiClemente, C., and Prochaska—
Transtheoretical Model Stages of
Change, 23, appC.232
diet, unhealthy, appA.155
dignity, in nurse coaching, 18,
23–24
diplomacy, in nurse coaching, 26
direct communication, appA.166–
168
disease-based model of care,
appA.144
disease management, appA.154–
155
disease prevention, appA.153
documentation, in nurse coaching,
13, 63–64, 66
Dossey, Barbara; Susan Luck; and
Bonney Gulino Schaub—Theory
of Integrative Nurse Coaching
(TINC), appB.223
Dossey, Barbara—Theory of Integral
Nursing (TIN), appB.219
doubt, in nurse coaching, 38

E

education, 13, 66, 81, appA. 141, appA. 171

educators, appA.136

elderly population, in nurse coaching, 43

electronic health records (EHRs), in nurse coaching, 13, 64, 66, appG.247–251

emotional intelligence, defined, appA.180

emotions, in nurse coaching, 14

empathy, in nurse coaching, 21, 33, 61

empirical knowing, app B. 216

empowerment
client-centered goals, appA.138

end-of-life care, in nurse coaching, 39

Enhanced Nurse Licensure Compact (eNLC) license, 25, 57

environment
defined, appA.180
external, appA.135, appA.140
healthy, appA.140
internal, appA.135, appA.140

environmental aspects of health, 13

environmental determinants of health, 10, appA.145
defined, appA.180

environmental ethics, in nurse coaching, 26, 35

environmental health, 5, 84, appA. 179, app H. 267

environmental risk factors, appA.147

Erickson, Helen; Evelyn Tomlin; and Mary Ann Swain—Theory of Modeling and Role Modeling (MRM), appA.209, appB.218–219

ethical knowing, app B. 216

ethics, 18, 26, 35, appA.135
competencies, 78–79, appA. 141, appA. 170, appH. 259–260
defined, appA.181

evaluation, 31, 32–33
competence, appA.144
competencies, 78, appA. 141, appA. 169, appH. 258–259
nurse coaching process, 78, appA.137
nursing process, appA.137, appA.141

evidence-based practice, 11, 13, 18, 53, 62
defined, appA.181

evidence-based practice and research, appA.146–147
competencies, 81, appA. 141, appH. 264–265 appA.172

evidence-informed practice, 18

evidence/research/theory, use of, appA.135

Executive Order 13548, appA.157

external environment, 19, appA.135, appA.140

F

families, in nurse coaching, 14, 20, 24, 39

fatigue, in nurse coaching, 30

Fawcett, J., appB.215

fear, in nurse coaching, 14

Federal Interagency Workgroup (FIW), appA.155

feelings, in nurse coaching, 30

findings, in nurse coaching, 39

fitness centers, in nurse coaching, 41

five structures of integral consciousness (Gebser), 22, appC.226–227

flexible spending account (FSA), 58

Fredrikson, B., appC.229

from novice to expert (Benner), appA.149

frustration, in nurse coaching, 14

The Future of Nursing (IOM report), appA.150

G

Gebser, J.,—five structures of integral consciousness, 22, appC.226–227

Gen X generation, 68

Gen Z generation, 68

goals, in nurse coaching, 10

governing organizations, in nurse coaching, 14

graduate and advanced practice nurse coach, competencies

assessment, appH.253–254

collaboration, appH.262

communication, appH.261

coordination of care, appH.258

culturally congruent practice, appH.260–261

diagnosis, appH.255

education, appH.263–264

environmental health, appH.267

ethics, appH.259–260

evaluation, appH.258–259

evidence-based practice and research, appH.264–265

implementation, appH.257–258

leadership, appH.262–263

outcome identification, appH.255–256

planning, appH.256–257

professional practice evaluation, appH.265–266

quality of practice, appH.265

resource utilization, appH.266–267

graduate coursework, in nurse coaching, 48, 52

grief, in nurse coaching, 38

groups, in nurse coaching, 14, 24, 36, 39, 42–43

growth, appA.148. *See also* self-healing

guidelines in nurse coaching, 14

The Guide to the Code of Ethics for Nurses with Interpretive Statements: Development, Interpretation, and Application, 23

H

harassment, in nurse coaching, 45

healing, 14, 20–21

defined, appA.181

healing intention

defined, appA.181

healing process

defined, appA.181

healing relationships

defined, appA.181

health

defined, appA.181

environmental determinants, appA.145

social determinants, 10, appA.145

Health and Human Services (HHS), appA.156

health and wellness programs, appA.148

health and wellness promotion model, appA.144

health as expanding consciousness theory (Neuman), 22, appA.205, appA.209–210, appB.220

health belief model (Becker), 22, appC.227–228

health beliefs, nurse coaching, 18

healthcare consumers, 14

coaching relationship with, 12

defined, 10

insurance, for nurse coaching, 57–59
integral, defined, appA.182
integral consciousness, appC.226
integral perspectives, 14, appA.146
integral theory, appA.149
integrative, defined, appA.182
integrative functional health model, appA.149
Integrative Health Policy Consortium (IHPC), 69
integrative knowing, appA.146
Integrative Nurse Coach Certificate Program (INCCP), appA.149
integrative perspectives, in nurse coaching, 14
integrity, in nurse coaching, 18, 26–27
intention, in nurse coaching, 19
interactions, coaching. *See* coaching interactions
interdisciplinary teams, in nurse coaching, 36
internal environment, 19, appA.135, appA.140
International Council of Nurses (ICN), 45, appA.149
internet-connected devices, in nurse coaching, 64
interprofessional collaboration, 13, 26, appA.151
interprofessional collaborative practice (IPCP), 47
interprofessional communications, 11
Interprofessional Internet Consultation, 66
interprofessional teams, 47–48
   high-performing, 47–48
   professional nurse coach, 11
   research, 39
intervention scheme, 63

intrapersonal dynamics, appA.151
intrinsic motivation, appC.226–227
intuition, defined, appA.182
irritability, in nurse coaching, 43
isolation, in nurse coaching, 43

J

job satisfaction, in nurse coaching, 56
judgments, in nurse coaching, 30
Jung, Carl, appC.231

K

Kauffman, C., appC.230
Kegan and Lahey—Immunity to Change, 22, appA.210, appC.228–229
knowing participation in change theory (Barrett), 22, appA.205, appA.208, appB.221–222
knowledge, in nurse coaching, 14, 38, 48, 59, 66

L

Lahey, L.L., and Kegan—Immunity to Change, 22, appA.210, appC.228–229
language, relevant use of, appA.166
leadership, 60–62, appA.153
   competencies, 80, appA.141, appA.175, appH.262–263
   nurse coaches role, appA.145
learning, 15, 25, 30, 38, 60, appA.143
   continuous, appA.154
Leihr, Patricia. *See* Smith, Jane Mary and Patricia Liehr
Leininger, Madeleine—Theory of Transcultural Nursing, appB.220–221

licenses, in nurse coaching, 57, 65, 66

life expectancy, in US, 54

lifelong personal learning, in nurse coaching, 15, 25

lifestyle, 30, 50, 54
    medicine, appA.154

listening, in nurse coaching, 15, 16, 32, 33, 34, 37, 40–41, 60, 66

literature search, in nurse coaching, 62

loneliness, in nurse coaching, 43

M

manageability, appC.233

Maslow, A., appC.230

Medicaid, 58, 65

Medicare, 58, 65

metaparadigm, in nursing theory, 17

millennial generation, 68

Mishel, Merle H.—Theory of Uncertainty in Illness (UIT), 22, appB.221–222

monitoring, in nurse coaching, 65

moral intelligence, defined, appA.182

mortality
    causes of, appA.155

motivation
    client-centered goals, 22, appA.138

motivational interviewing (Miller and Rollnick), 23, appC.228–229

motivations, in nurse coaching, 16

multiple sclerosis, in nurse coaching, 54

Munhall, P.L., app B.215

N

National Center for Healthcare Leadership (NCHL), 46, 61

National Committee on Quality Care (NCQA), 58

National Consortium for the Credentialing of Health and Wellness Coaches (NCCHWC), appA.144, appA.151

National Council on State Boards of Nursing (NCSBN), 65

National Institute of Health, 62

National Prevention Strategy, appA.155, appA.156–157

national provider identification (NPI) number, 58

NCCHWC. *See* National Consortium for the Credentialing of Health and Wellness Coaches (NCCHWC)

needs, in nurse coaching, 34

neighborhood revitalization initiative, appA.157

Neuman, Betty—Neuman Systems Model (NSM), app B.217–218 app B.217–218

Newman, Margaret—Health as Expanding Consciousness Theory, 11, 22, appA.209, appB. 220

Nightingale, F., 36, appA.145–146
    nurse theorist, appA.145–146

Notes on Hospitals (Nightingale), 36

Notes on Nursing (Nightingale), 36

not-knowing, app B. 216
    defined, appA.182

nurse coach–client relationship, appA.139, appA.146, appA.148, appA.151

nurse coach(es)
    in clinical settings, 40–41
    communication, 33–34
    community health programs, 44–45
    cultural care, 36–37
    defined, appA.183
    descriptive characteristics, 40
    education, 38

professional nurse coach performance competencies. *See competencies.*

professional trends and issues
    health and healthcare in the United States, 54–55
    nurse coaching workforce, 55–57

protocols, in nurse coaching, 14

psychiatric and non-psychiatric settings, in nurse coaching, 46

psychological aspects, nurse coaching
    of health, 13

psychosynthesis (Assagioli), 23, appC.230

public policy, in nurse coaching, 18

Q

qualitative method, in nurse coaching, 14

quality of care, in nurse coaching, 41

quality of practice
    competencies, 81–82, appA. 141, appA.173, appH. 265

quantitative method, in nurse coaching, 14

R

recertification, in nurse coaching, 52

referrals, appA.153

reflective practices (Johns), 23, appC.232–233

registered nurses (RNs), nurse coaching, 17, 47, 51

regulations, in nurse coaching, 25, 57

regulatory organizations, in nurse coaching, 14

reimbursement, for nurse coaching, 57–59

relational coordination, in nurse coaching, 47

relationship, 14, 31, 48
    relationship-centered caring process, 31–32
    relationship-centered coaching, appA.135, appA.139

relevant use of language, appA.166

religion, in nurse coaching, 24

research, 14, 26, 39, 62, appA.146

resilience (Polk), 14, 23, appC.233

Resnick, Barbara—Theory of Self-Efficacy, 22, appB.223

resource utilization
    competencies, 26, 84, appA.142, appH. 266–267, appA.178

respect, in nurse coaching, 15, 18, 19, 21, 23–24, 35, 48

responsibility, in nurse coaching, 15, 25

rights, in nurse coaching, 24–25

rituals, in nurse coaching, 37, 38

Robert Wood Johnson Foundation (RWJF), appA.150

Rogers, Martha—Theory of Science of Unitary Human Beings, appB.219, appC.231

role delineation study (RDS), 5

Roy, Callista—Roy Adaptation Model, appA.207, appB.217

Ryan, Richard and Edward Deci—self-determination theory, 22, appC.227

S

safety, in nurse coaching, 24–25

scholarly inquiry, in nurse coaching, 26

science and art, incorporation of, appA.135

Sebelius, K., appA.156
secondary traumatic stress (STS), in nurse coaching, 47
self-assessment, 30, 53, appA.143, appA.152
self-awareness, 15, appA.147, appA.148, appA.152
self-care, 11, 15, 44, appA.143, appA.149, appA.152
Self-Care Deficit Nursing Theory (Orem), 21, appA.148, appA.206, appB.218
self-care model, of nursing, appA.148
self-centeredness, in nurse coaching, 43
self-defeating patterns, in nurse coaching, 15
self-determination theory (SDT), 22, appC.227
self-development, 15, appA.136, appA.143, appA.152, appA.154
activities, appA.154
self-discovery, appA.135
self-efficacy (Bandura), 23, 33, 66, appC.234
self-esteem, in nurse coaching, 33
self-evaluation, 30, appA.143, appA.152
self-healing, 14, appA.148, appA.151
self–knowledge, appA.148
self-rated depression scale (SDS), 44, 45
self-reflection, 15, appA.143, appA.152
Seligman, Martin and Mihaly Csikszentmihalyi—Positive Psychology, 23, appA.135, appA.211, appC.230
sense-of-coherence theory (SOC), 23, appC.233–234
sense of presence, in nurse coaching, 15

sensors, in nurse coaching, 64
sexual orientation, in nurse coaching, 18, 24
shame, in nurse coaching, 38
Sigma Theta Tau International (STTI), appA.149
skills, in nurse coaching, 38, 66
sleep disorders, in nurse coaching, 45, 46
Smith, Marlaine—Theory of Unitary Caring, appB.222
Smith, Mary Jane and Patricia Liehr—Story Theory, appB.222
smoking, mortality and morbidity, 54
social contract, 2
social determinants, health, 10, appA.145
social justice, in nurse coaching, 18, 26–27
social responsibility, 2
social sciences, appA.144
social structures, in nurse coaching, 37
social support theory, appA.149
socio-economic status, in nurse coaching, 24
sociological aspects, nurse coaching, 13
sociopolitical knowing, app B. 216–217
specialties, in nurse coaching, 39, 44
spiritual beliefs in nurse coaching, 13, 24
staff nurses, 39, appA.136
Standards of Practice, 4–5, 19–20, appA.140–142, appA.150, appA. 159–169
Standards of Professional Performance, 3–5, 19, appA. 140–142, appA. 170–179

statutes, in nurse coaching, 57

story theory (Smith and Leihr), 22 appA.205, appB.222

stress, in nurse coaching, 45, 47

stress management programs, in nurse coaching, 44

stress related illnesses, appA.147

substance use disorder, in nurse coaching, 54

suffering, in nurse coaching, 15

suicide rate, in US, 54

symbols, in nurse coaching, 37

systems model (Neuman), 21, appB.217–218

systolic blood pressure (SBP), 44, 45

T

T'ai Chi, 43

technology, in nurse coaching, 66

telephone, in nurse coaching, 65–66

The Ever Present Origin (Jean Gebser), appC.226

theory-guided practice, in nurse coaching, 13

theory of human becoming (Parse), 22, appA.205, appA.208, appB.219–220

theory of human caring and care science (Watson). *See Watson, Jean Theory of Transpersonal Caring/ Unitary Caring Science*

theory of integral nursing (Dossey), 21, appB.219

theory of integrative nurse coaching (Dossey, Luck, and Schaub), 22, appB.223

theory of interpersonal relations, 22, appA.148, appB.221

theory of interpersonal relations (Peplau), appA.148, appB.221

theory of modeling and role-modeling (Erickson, Tomlin, and Swain), 21, appA.209, appB.218–219

theory of science of unitary human beings (Rogers), 22, appB.219, appC.223

theory of self-efficacy (Resnick), 22, appB.223

theory of transcultural nursing (Leininger), 22, appB.220

theory of transpersonal caring and caring science, appC.231

theory of uncertainty in illness (Mishel), 22, appB.221–222

theory of unitary caring (Smith), 22, appB.222

theory of unitary human beings, appC.231

therapeutic partnerships, appA.149

the transtheoretical model (TTM), appC.231–232

threats, in nurse coaching, 45

tobacco use, appA.155

training, in nurse coaching, 13, 66

transpersonal, defined, appA.154

transpersonal psychology (Grof), 23, appC.230–231

transtheoretical model stages of change (Prochaska and DiClemente), 23, appC.232

triple/quadruple aim, 11

trust, in nurse coaching, 19, 21, 38, 60

U

uncertainty, in nurse coaching, 38

unhealthy diet, appA.155

unitary appreciative inquiry (Cowling), 22, appA.210, appB.223

unitary knowing in nursing practice (Cowling), 22. appB.220

United States
statistical snapshot, appA.144–155
U.S. Department of Health and Human Services (HHS), 67, appA.156

V

values, in nurse coaching, 10, 12, 18, 30, 37

verbal and nonverbal information, in nurse coaching, 33, 34

violence, in nurse coaching, 25, 34, 45–46, 61

vulnerability model (Schaub and Schaub), 23, appA.149, appC.234–235

W

Watson, Jean, appA.123, appA.124
caritas coaching program, appA.149

Theory of Transpersonal Caring/ Unitary Caring Science, 22, appA.205, appA.209, appB.221

theory of transpersonal caring and caring science, appC.231

wearable devices, in nurse coaching, 64

well-being, appA.140

White, J., app B.215

Whitney, D., appC.225

WHO. *See* World Health Organization (WHO)

workplace
creating healthy culture, 46
support for healthy, 47
violence and incivility, 45–46, 61

World Health Organization (WHO), 47, appA.155

worth, in nurse coaching, 23–24

Y

YMCAs, in nurse coaching, 41

yoga, 43